Voices from the
Prostate Underground

Voices from the Prostate Underground

✦

Dave Pratt

iUniverse, Inc.
New York   Bloomington

Voices from the Prostate Underground

Copyright © 2008 by Dave Pratt

iUniverse books may be ordered through booksellers or by contacting:

iUniverse
1663 Liberty Drive
Bloomington, IN 47403
www.iuniverse.com
1-800-Authors (1-800-288-4677)

ISBN: 978-1-4401-0148-9 (pbk)
ISBN: 978-1-4401-0149-6 (ebk)

Printed in the United States of America

iUniverse Rev. Date 11/18/08

Foreword

There's no easy way to get the news that you have cancer, whether it is prostate cancer, breast cancer, or any other type. Most logic and rational thought processes you have used in the past go out the window as you wrestle with a disease that carries such frightening connotations. Mention the word *cancer* to your friends and family and watch their responses. They become awkward, over react, and simply won't know what to do with the news. The very people who want to be there for you at that very difficult time will not be able to relate.

The good news is that you are not alone and there is a lot to be hopeful about. A lot of us have been down that road, and every day, medical studies and anecdotal evidence suggest that prostate cancer, in specific, has a very good survival rate when diagnosed and treated early.

Prostate cancer and the men who have wrestled with its effects are what this book is all about. Men are diagnosed with prostate cancer at a rate of more than 200,000 a year. Some 30,000 will die of the disease each year. The good news is that the disease can be detected with simple tests such as the PSA (prostate specific antigen) and DRE (digital rectal exam), which are referred to by prostate cancer experts as generally effective diagnostic tools. More good news is the growing arsenal of weapons that the medical field has to fight the disease.

The bad news is that men don't seem to want to talk about prostate cancer. It's just not done. There is something about the disease that seems to threaten our masculinity. That perception probably has to do with the traditionally accepted forms of treatment for the disease, and the relatively high rates of impotence and incontinence associated with those treatments. One of the last things a fifty year-old man wants to deal with is impotence or the possibility of wearing diapers for the rest of his life.

Treatment for prostate cancer comes in numerous varieties. When I was diagnosed, there were half a dozen treatments that had a high likelihood of curing my cancer. Unfortunately, few doctors are aware of all the treatment types and too often limit their recommendations to only those that they personally can carry out. The patient does not get the benefit of exposure to other, equally effective forms of treatment that may impact their post-treatment quality of life to greater or lesser degrees.

The stories in this book are provided by men and their wives, told in their own voices, who have gone through prostate cancer and its treatment. Each has wrestled with the issues of the cancer, making the best decision they could, considering their access to care, the advice they received. In most cases, the outcomes of their decisions have been very good.

There are stories from men whose cancer was caught early and the results were highly satisfactory. One man was pronounced terminal by his doctor, with only three months to live. He submitted his story for this book seventeen years later, while living a full and active life. In every case, these men and their wives took charge of their disease and its treatment, and that has made all the difference. My thanks go out to all those who submitted their stories for this book. They are the voices from the Prostate Underground.

If you have prostate cancer, be sure that you see your physician and work with him or her to determine the best course of treatment for your situation. As you do that, understand that it is you who must be the "patient warrior"; the one who leads the attack against your cancer. Your doctor, your wife, and the rest of your support team can help you along your journey, but the responsibility for treatment is yours and yours alone. I hope these stories help as you deal with the decisions you have to make along the way.

Nothing in this book is intended as medical advice, nor should it be taken that way. The stories are provided by men and their wives who have dealt with prostate cancer. The stories are provided as examples of how others have wrestled with their disease and come to terms with it. In many cases, they lived long lives in spite of initial diagnoses to the contrary.

As with disease of any kind, if you think you might have prostate cancer, be sure to talk to your doctor immediately. Seek medical advice and treatment. Do it early. Do it now.

I hope that the stories contained in this book, provided in the cancer survivors' own words, provide you with some insight and hope. Remember that no matter what anyone tells you to the contrary, there is always hope.

You can survive prostate cancer.

Contents

Stories from the Prostate Underground

Dave from Yelm – Proton Beam

HOW THE JOURNEY BEGAN

There isn't any good way to learn that you have cancer.

In my case, the day already wasn't going so well. Our new puppy had broken its toe, was in a cast and driving the household crazy. It was like Tiny Tim on steroids; a cute little peg-leg creature clumping around the hardwood floors, tearing up shoes, newspapers and anything else within reach.

Then the doctor called.

The results of my recent physical exam were in. "Your PSA score is high. That measures your Prostate Specific Antigen," he said. He seemed to have ruled out an enlarged prostate or infection, so that left one other choice.

"I need you to come into the office. I need to do a biopsy to check for cancer," he said.

The mind went numb at the c-word. I thanked the doctor even as he continued to talk, and hung up the phone.

My wife entered the room as the phone rang again. This time she picked it up. She listened for a few minutes and I distantly heard her say, "Thank you, Doctor. We'll see you at your office next week. No, I'm sure he didn't mean to hang up on you like that. Goodbye."

My wife handled the news with a lot of cool. However, cool was not a factor for me. I felt cold, numb, and it was a sensation that endures.

This sort of scenario is played out nearly 200,000 times a year. Around 30,000 men die from prostate cancer each year. Even so, the issues and facts related to prostate cancer are not front-page news, and sometimes are hard to find. This, in spite of the fact that prostate cancer has a high cure rate when caught early.

Jim Keifert, a seventeen-year cancer survivor and active in Us TOO, an international men's prostate cancer support group, summed it up by saying, "Prostate cancer is perceived as something that attacks a man's masculinity. Guys don't like to talk about it, so the message doesn't get out."

When my own urologist completed my biopsy and confirmed that I did in fact have cancer, the next words out of his mouth were, "Let's get you scheduled for surgery."

When you are diagnosed with cancer, you become very vulnerable. You feel like your body is out of control. What you want most is for someone to just make it go away. I was only too happy to agree to the surgery.

Shortly after that, a good friend called and said, "Don't agree to surgery until you talk to my friend. He went through what you're going through and had a great treatment that doesn't have the side effects of surgery."

Five minutes later his friend called me from back east. During our conversation, he advised me of a key point that my urologist left out of our earlier discussion: There were at least five types of treatment available to me. Surgery wasn't the only option. All had about the same chance for a cure.

I called my urologist and asked about one of those treatments, called Proton Therapy. During some quick research, I discovered that the treatment has been used effectively for over 14,000 patients at one facility.

"It's a gimmick," he said. "The best answer for you is cold hard steel."

Those were his exact words, and they just didn't sit right with me. It was enough to motivate me to research further.

Jim Keifert summed up the situation by saying, "Surgeons know surgery. Your urologist has confidence in his skill as a surgeon, so he recommended that. A radiation oncologist might recommend radiation therapy, since that's what he or she is most familiar with. Each approach may well work. The bottom line is that it's up to you to select the best treatment for your situation."

For the next four weeks, I researched prostate cancer treatment. I talked with two radiation oncologists, two urologists, a host of other healthcare professionals, and visited countless websites on the Internet.

The upshot of that effort was that, given my type and severity of cancer, I did indeed have five or more treatment options. The good news was that each form of treatment promised approximately the same level of success, even though the side effects varied. As one particularly enlightened urologist said, "The good news is that you have five choices for treatment. The bad news is you have five choices for treatment.

Now, I had to make a choice.

We men are our own worst enemies when it comes to prostate cancer. We simply don't talk about it, because of the perceived threat to our masculinity. The information is actually fairly abundant, but exists within a close knit group of survivors and enlightened physicians, a sort of Prostate Underground who help other men with their prostate cancer, while not making it too public.

NEXT STEPS

Bringing up a new puppy and being diagnosed with prostate cancer may seem like two separate issues, but put a cast on that little dog and a strange sort of metaphor evolves.

Smudge, our Schipperke puppy, broke a toe. When we took him to the vet, she put him in a cast and predicted a two-week recovery. If you think raising a puppy in a cast is no big deal, try house-breaking a dog in a cast. Fourteen days can be a very long time for both the carpets and a person's sanity

Two weeks later, we returned to the vet. "It looks fine," she said. "We'll just leave this cast on for a couple more weeks to be sure."

We gritted our teeth, accepting that Tiny Tim on steroids would be with us for a while longer. However, at the end of the next two weeks, when an additional fortnight was prescribed, our frustration peaked. The dog was driving us crazy, thumping around the hardwood floor and paddling his cast in the water bowl. Was a full six weeks in a cast really necessary?

We were certain the vet is trying to do the best thing for the puppy, but how are we to know what is right or what is wrong when it comes to treating broken puppy toes?

The same could be said for finding the best way to treat prostate cancer.

After the obligatory biopsy, prostate cancer is generally evaluated in terms of a Gleason Score. Gleason rates the cancer in terms of aggressiveness, along a scale from 1 to 10. My Gleason was 6. According to my doctor, 7 was the dividing line between aggressive and non-aggressive cancer. Good news.

The next step was a physical exam. From that, the cancer was graded based on the presence or absence of nodules and signs of spreading. My grade was a T-1-c. This was a good score. No nodules were found and it looked like the cancer wasn't spreading outside the prostate.

It was my lucky day. If we had been talking about anything other than cancer, I might have cheered.

After getting the good news, I started digging into the information about prostate cancer and its treatment. My urologists' opinion was clear: "cold hard steel" was my best option. Those were his exact words, although the side effects of a radical prostatectomy, such as impotence, incontinence and urethral blockage, did not appeal to me. There had to be other options.

As it turns out, there were. The list was fairly extensive, including robotic assisted laparoscopic prostatectomy, hormone therapy, external beam radiation, proton therapy, brachytherapy, and more.

However, after weeks of digging, I could find nothing to suggest how a person should select the best form of treatment for prostate cancer. Simply put, there were no clinical studies that showed the effects and outcomes of different types of treatment. It was like all the really important information had disappeared into some sort of Prostate Underground.

For help, I contacted Dr. Paul Lange, Chief of the Urology Department at the University of Washington Medical Center, and a prostate cancer survivor. "Why isn't there any information about how to choose the best form of treatment?" I asked.

According to Lange, most Americans do not see themselves as a participant in the solution when it comes to their health. In our culture, Lang explains, we have not accepted the idea of the "patient as warrior

Did he have any advice for a person my age, with my cancer "numbers"?

His response was surprising, especially coming from a urologist who has done over 2,000 prostate surgeries and is a leader in his field. At my age and with my Gleason, Lang did not recommend surgery. "Unless the person has a psychological need to remove the tissue from the body," he offered. First, he suggested, I should look at the many other good options.

So, I made two very important decisions.

First, the puppy's cast comes off this week. Second, in two weeks I head to Loma Linda Medical Center to start Proton Therapy. The puppy can finally be house-broken and I can deal with this cancer. There are no guarantees, either with housebreaking or cancer, but the decision felt right, and I suppose that's the best anyone can do.

TREATMENT CHOICES AND PERSONAL OUTCOMES

I was diagnosed with prostate cancer and my Schipperke puppy broke its toe at about the same time. The decision on what to do about the pup was a no-brainer. You take the dog to your local vet and they do what's needed. Picking the best way to treat my cancer was another matter, altogether.

There are a variety of treatments available to treat and cure prostate cancer, and for a person with my type of cancer they all do about the same good job. Whether it's surgery, radiation, cryosurgery, or brachytherapy, the outcomes are about the same. It's when I researched the side effects of the treatments that the differences became apparent, and caused me the most concern.

A study by Doctors Bhatnagar and Kaplan a few years ago compared the side effects of the various forms of prostate cancer treatment and found striking differences. Surgical removal of the prostate carried up to a 17% risk of bowel dysfunction, 90% risk of impotence, and up to a 60% chance of urinary incontinence. Traditional radiation treatment resulted in a 30% risk bowel dysfunction, an 85% risk of impotence, and a 30% risk of urinary incontinence.

At 53 years old, I was not enamored by the prospect of impotence or having to wear a diaper. I set out to find another alternative, and that's when, with the help of some close friends, I discovered Proton Therapy.

Proton Therapy is different from traditional radiation, which relies on photons to kill the cancer. In traditional radiation therapy, "photons" are shot at the cancer and discharge their energy on the way to the target. They lose a lot of their energy and damage the tissue on the way to, around and through the target. The photon beam then continues out the other side of the body. This accompanying tissue damage accounts for many of the side effects commonly associated with photon beam radiation.

In Proton Therapy, "protons" are shot at the target. Because of their unique characteristics, they discharge their energy at the cancer target. The beam does very little damage on the way in, then stops at the target and, unlike photon radiation, does not continue on through the body. Proton beams can be very accurately targeted using three dimensional imaging, so damage to surrounding tissue and organs is a lot less likely, although it can happen.

Dr. James Metz of the University of Pennsylvania Cancer Center compared proton cancer treatment to other forms of treatment and found the risk of long-term impotence to be less than 30%, urinary incontinence at less than 1%, and colon dysfunction at near zero.

When I saw those figures, I felt like I'd found my answer. When I talked to a dozen or so patients who'd received Proton Therapy over the past sixteen years, I was sold. There are still risks, but they seem a lot less than the alternatives.

After two weeks, I started treatment at Loma Linda. My treatment lasted about 60 days, during which time I lived in California near the medical center. If there was a drawback to the treatment, it was that I had to be near the hospital for that long a time so I could be treated five days a week for 44 treatments. On the other hand, I'm 53 years old. My life expectancy is about 30 years, or 10,000 days. The 60 days it took for my treatment seemed pretty small compared to the 10,000 days I stood to gain.

As a side note, Smudge, the puppy did well. His leg was malformed from being in a cast for so long during his formative years, but even that seems to be coming around.

FAMILY, FRIENDS AND SUPPORT GROUPS

When our three month-old Schipperke puppy, Smudge, broke his foot and was put in a cast, my wife and I immediately moved into patient support mode. We coddled the dog, going out of our way to make him comfortable.

The strange thing was, Smudge didn't seem to appreciate the coddling. Instead, he wanted to continue to play ball and steal my wife's socks like he did before his foot was in a cast. We went with the flow, chasing after him when he stole something and tossing the ball while he did a credible impression of Charles Dickens' Tiny Tim as he thumped around the house in his puppy-sized splint.

Smudge's foot healed over time and he's grown into an apparently healthy, happy, larger version of the sock-stealer he was before the injury. I have to think that's a good thing, even if the socks do suffer.

I was diagnosed with prostate cancer about the same time Smudge broke his foot. Like Smudge, when I got the news the last thing I wanted was coddling. In fact, whenever someone approached me in that manner, I withdrew and even pushed back. I built an emotional wall around me to avoid that sort of treatment by others.

Thank goodness I went to a place for my treatment where coddling and emotional isolation isn't on the agenda, where the focus is on patient support and seeing a little humor in every situation.

Effective patient support and humor have, in fact, been shown to have a positive effect on cancer patients and their treatment. At Loma Linda University Medical Center, where I receive Proton Therapy, there are no less than three support group meetings/pot luck dinners each week. During the largest of those, 100 to 160 men attend. Most have prostate cancer, and all can be heard listening to or telling jokes, exchanging experiences and supporting each other. The mood is light and always positive. To a man, attendees continually remark about the positive impact the gathering has on them during their time at Loma Linda.

Bringing that many men together to share their experiences may sound like an odd sort of gathering, but there is actual research that shows that support groups have a positive impact on cancer patients. A study by Vicki S. Helgeson and Sheldon Cohen of Carnegie Mellon University showed that participation in support groups made up of others with cancer enhanced patient self-esteem, restored a sense of perceived control, and instilled a sense of optimism.

Believe me, when you're told you have cancer, you feel lower than low. The world seems out of control and optimism is very hard to come by. Borrowing a little self esteem, sense of control, and positive attitude from others with my same condition in a support group has been a very big help in adapting to my situation.

And what about all the joking around that we do when we're together at the support group?

Dr. Lee Berk of the Department of Pathology at the Loma Linda School of Medicine has been studying the effects of laughter on cancer and the immune system for years. He and his peers have found that laughter, for example, increases the number and activity of natural killer cells in the body, the cells that attack virus and tumor cells. "The mind and body are inherently linked. Laughter is a strong tool in our battle against cancer and other diseases," said Dr. Berk during our recent interview.

I suspect that Smudge and I both enjoyed a good laugh. His innate cheerfulness was probably why the pup's foot healed so quickly. It was also why I was positive about my chances for a cure. I laughed at the thought of Smudge charging around the house with one of my wife's socks in his mouth. It made my day, even if is hard on the socks. I laughed at the jokes at our support group and I just seemed a bit better.

If you're someone with cancer, think about joining a support group. If you have prostate cancer, check out UsTOO. They meet in many locations around the world. If you go to a meeting, don't forget to take a good joke.

LIFE GOES ON

When my Schipperke puppy, Smudge, broke his toe and recovered from that injury, there was little question about what he'd do with the rest of his life. There were bones to chew, flowers to dig up, strangers to bark at, books to steal off shelves, and the other dogs in the house to terrorize. When the cast came off, he simply picked up where he left off, although with a level of intensity that was missing during the six weeks he spent in a splint.

For me, diagnosed with prostate cancer at about the same time as Smudge broke his toe and about to complete my treatments, the question of what lies ahead seems a bit more complex. As I approached the last few weeks of a treatment, it seemed like I had been doubly blessed. Through the help of good friends, I found a treatment that has a good chance of curing my cancer. Ands of the date when I wrote this, my PSA had dropped to 0.87, which was right on target. I was given the chance to do something with my life, things that I might not have been able to do if my cancer had gone untreated.

What do you do with your life after you've made it through a life-threatening trial like cancer?

I put the question to other patients who have received, or are receiving, treatment for prostate cancer. Some continued the battle by helping others fight the disease, such as Dan, from St. Louis. "I became a very active patient advocate.

For the past three years, I have been a patient advocate on Cancer and Leukemia Group B, one of (the National Cancer Institute's) cooperative research groups." With the help of one of his local hospitals, Dan started a prostate cancer support group in which he remains active.

Other prostate cancer survivors felt it was enough to return to their lives as they were before they contracted the disease. This was enough for Robert from Pittsburgh, who said, "The impact of the cancer has affected me psychologically. I have become a little overly sensitive to every ache and pain (I call them the ache and pain of the week). On the other hand, my professional life was really not impacted. As a professor, I have continued to meet my students' and professional obligations. In fact, a year after my treatment, I took my class to Germany for a special Spring Break program."

These two men have very different outlooks on how their lives should be after cancer. Both are courageous individuals who have braved one of the most fearsome opponents a person can come up against.

So, what will I do?

I think I'll listen to both men. As Dr. J. Lynn Martell, leader of Loma Linda's Radiation Medicine/Education Support Group so often says, "We want our patients to go back to their lives, live those lives and be able to put their cancer behind them." Robert took that approach, and it worked for him.

On the other hand, the Prostate Cancer Underground is very much a reality. The public and those who have had the disease still are generally not talking. When they do talk, it's from a variety of confusing perspectives. The wide variety of treatment options available to men with the disease, and the fact that all too often family physicians, urologists and oncologists are not aware of those options, makes in imperative that the information gets out so that those with prostate cancer can make a reasoned approach to their treatment options.

Like Robert, I wanted to get on with my life. Like Dan, I thought that getting the word out about treatment options and helping others fight cancer seemed like a good option. I hope this book goes a little ways toward continuing the fight.

Dan from St. Louis – Surgery

HOW THE JOURNEY BEGAN

My father had died of advanced prostate cancer in 1982. I had the same urologist for an unrelated kidney condition and when I went to see him, he said there was a new blood test he'd like me to have. A few days later my wife called and asked if I could meet her for lunch. She had never done that before, so I suspected something was afoot.

We had received a letter from my doctor, she informed me at lunch. My PSA (prostate specific antigen), the doctor's letter said, was a little high: 8-something. That was back in 1990 and subsequent, periodic ultrasound biopsies were negative, meaning that there was no cancer. Already, I was beginning to learn the cancer lingo, where negative is positive, and positive is a bad thing.

Little did I know how things would change.

NEXT STEPS

In the summer of 1992, my wife said she thought we should get a second opinion, since the PSA continued to be at 8 or 9. The urologist we saw did a biopsy and found two positive biopsy samples out of seven, with a Gleason Score of 2+2, or 4. That doctor was in Saint Louis, and my wife and I decided on a radical prostatectomy after she called the NCI 1-800-4-cancer line and got more information than I wanted to think about.

We told our two daughters, my law partner, my secretary and some good friends who lived in Saint Louis. I did not tell my mother. I did not want to worry her, since she was 92 and I was concerned if she learned I had the "Big C", it might adversely affect her.

TREATMENT CHOICES AND PERSONAL OUTCOMES

I chose surgery. It went well, except for the sad coincidence that my mother suffered a cerebral hemorrhage and died while I was recovering in Saint Louis. Jewish Hospital (since merged into Barnes-Jewish), where I was treated, was an excellent hospital. One male nurse on the night shift was especially helpful, as was a female nurse who brought me through the first day.

My urologist was very helpful, as were the residents who often came with him to see me. The only thing he didn't prepare me for was what came after the surgery: sexual orgasms would be dry. That may not be too bad a thing at age 64, but it was weird and unexpected.

FAMILY, FRIENDS AND SUPPORT GROUPS

My family was all very supportive. One of the daughters took time from her work and family in Austin, Texas to come be with my wife and me for the surgery and a few days afterward. Our Saint Louis friends were supportive, too, and visited me at the hospital and then we went to their house for a few days before returning home.

My wife was wonderfully supportive all through the experience, and has been since. My law firm, when I got back to the office and started lawyering again, also helped with my transition. I was back on my feet in just three and a half weeks, so all the support made it easy for me.

The funniest thing that happened was when my urologist gave me my initial injection of what was one of the early erectile dysfunction drugs, one he actually had to get from the Children's Hospital, because it wasn't yet being marketed for erectile dysfunction. We left his office and it took dramatic effect as I was driving home. That was a bit uncomfortable.

LIFE GOES ON

The big change was really in that I became a very active patient advocate. For the past three years I have been a patient advocate for Cancer and Leukemia Group B, one of NCI's cooperative research groups. The other area in which I still spend time is with our local Us TOO support group.

With the help of one of our local hospitals, I started a prostate cancer support group, in which I remain active. It would have been helpful during my decision process, I'm sure, but even had there been one in my town then, I wouldn't have taken advantage of it because of my desire to keep it under wraps.

I wasn't as sold on the value of humor in treatment of cancer then as I am now. A good attitude plays a big role in things.

I had read a Norman Cussins book and one of Bernie Siegal's books, and as a result, a primary aid to my recovery came through relaxation response training and self-hypnosis, that I learned from a book and audio tape that I got from our local library. I used the techniques before and after my surgery and felt it was very helpful.

After surgery when the post-op pathology showed possibly unclean margins, I developed a cheer for my healing system that I continue to use today:

> "Healing system, do your stuff. Chase cancer
> cells and treat 'em rough. When we get done,
> they'll know what hit 'em. Then we'll p---
> 'em out or s--- 'em"

As the surgeon suspected, the pathology was apparently an artifact of the surgery and as the PSA remained undetectable, I decided to forego the possibility of adjuvant radiation therapy to the prostate bed.

Paul from Las Vegas – Proton Beam

How the Journey Began

(Comments are from Paul's wife.)

This story began in June 2006 when Paul decided to go to the Veterans' Administration seeking "cheaper" medications. This turned out to be not worth the effort.

To make a long story short, the VA gave him a full set of blood tests. It turned out that his PSA (prostate specific antigen) had raised significantly, from 0.8 the previous reading in November 2005, so we went to see a urologist.

We refer to him as doctor #2. Doctor #1 didn't do much for us, and was not much more than a "blip on the radar. #2 did a nineteen core biopsy last August, which turned out to be negative. In January 2007 Paul had another PSA test, and it had risen again, to 0.9. Although the PSA was still in the "normal" range, the rate of increase was too high. We have since learned that this is a red flag in the world of prostate cancer.

Not wishing to give #2 another opportunity to miss anything that might be there, we took a 5+ hour trip to Ventura, California to see a well-known radiologist who specializes in color Doppler ultrasound targeted biopsies of the prostate. A targeted biopsy was taken and this time the results were positive.

On February 20, 2007, the California doctor personally called me and delivered the diagnosis of prostate cancer. He gave me the gory details of Gleason Score of 3 + 4, or 7, the percentage of each core that was positive, a stage based on a digital rectal exam (DRE), and some other information which I don't remember now. We thought we had caught it at a relatively early stage, but were not sure.

NEXT STEPS

Thus began a month of intense research into all the available treatment options. Doctor #3 (#2 is history at this point) said Paul was not a candidate for surgery, at least from his perspective, but that he was a candidate for various types of radiation treatment.

We considered seeds, both temporary and permanent, as well as external radiation guided by various methods. Over the period of a month, we met with one medical oncologist who specialized in prostate cancer and three radiation oncologists. In addition, we met with doctor #3 twice.

It was quite an education. On our first visit to doctor #3, we asked him about Loma Linda's Proton Therapy treatment for prostate cancer. He categorized Loma Linda as "smoke and mirrors".

On our second visit, he was quite supportive when we told him of our decision to go to Loma Linda University Medical Center, and asked if Paul still wanted him to be his urologist. He said that he had spoken to the other physicians we had consulted and the group consensus was that, from the questions we asked at each interview, we should be going to

Loma Linda. He also stated that "no money changed hands on the informal bets on what treatment option we would choose".

TREATMENT CHOICES AND PERSONAL OUTCOMES

On April 1, we headed to Loma Linda University Medical Center, in Loma Linda CA, for nine weeks of proton treatment. Proton therapy is a form of radiation which has been reported to have fewer side effects and is acknowledged by the physicians with whom we spoke to be as effective as other forms of radiation in treating prostate cancer. Paul has spoken to a number of men who have been through this treatment for prostate cancer at Loma Linda and all, without exception, report good results with few side effects. We hope to be part of that group.

As of this survey (23 treatments down and 19 to go) he has had very few and minor side effects. Paul is on Flomax and that has kept the urinary problems to a minimum. He has not had severe anything, fatigue, depression, weight loss, weight gain, etc.

FAMILY, FRIENDS AND SUPPORT GROUPS

Paul attended an US Too meeting in Las Vegas before we got to Loma Linda for treatment. He attended one Wednesday evening pep rally at Loma Linda when he was being prodded by his wife and others, and one when he started treatment. He felt he was not a support group type of guy. It is fine for those who need and enjoy that type of support, but he preferred informal chats with other patients, and things like the pot-lucks and Thursday restaurant meetings that the hospital sponsors for its patients.

LIFE GOES ON

Other than the costs of the co-pays and the staying in Loma Linda, there wasn't much impact on Paul. I remain very upset about the experience and expect that I will not get over this easily due to our circumstances. I am hopeful that the "Frying Time" I spent here does the job and that he will be disease free for many years. As Nancy, one of the radiation technicians used to say during treatment, "Is it soup yet?"

Now, we wait and see...

Clayton from Puyallup – Proton Beam

How the Journey Began

It all started with my annual physical on December 4, 2006. My doctor said my PSA count had increased from 2.3 to 3.3 in the last year. He explained that was too big of an increase and suggested I see a urologist for a urologic evaluation. Also he said he felt a hard place on my prostate. My doctor gave me the names of two Urologists he recommended.

I got an appointment with the first one on the list for December 21, 2006. At this examination, the rectal exam showed normal tone – no masses on the prostate – an indurated area at the right base, with no distinct nodule. The plan was to proceed with prostate ultrasound and biopsy. An appointment was made for January 3, 2007. The Urologist called me on January 5, 2007 and told me about the results and wanted me to come in January 8, 2007 at 4:00 PM to discuss the treatment options.

NEXT STEPS

At the January 8 visit the Urologist explained that I had a Gleason Score of 3+4=7, with more cancer on the right side than the left side. The clinical stage is B2, T2C. He then explained my options.

After thoughtful prayer and research I decided to look into Intensity Modulated Radiation Therapy (IMRT) and Laparoscopic Radical Prostatectomy (LRP). I made appointments with doctors in both areas for IMRT on January 15 and LRP on January 30.

My wife pulled the different options from the Internet. I did much reading, as well. Also did a lot of talking with family, friends and neighbors.

One neighbor knew a friend who went to California for treatments. Since I also knew this person, I called him and the next night he came to my house and we talked for one and a half hours. He had proton treatment at Loma Linda in 2002. He gave me the phone number to call to get an informational packet. I called the next morning and two days later had the packet. My wife also pulled information on proton therapy and Loma Linda University Medical Center from the Internet.

On January 15, 2007 I visited a Radiation Oncology Center and had a consultation with a doctor. He recommended me as a good candidate for any of the treatment options including Prostatectomy, External Beam Radiation Therapy with IMRT, with or with out Radioactive Seeds implant or Radioactive Seeds implant alone.

TREATMENT CHOICES AND PERSONAL OUTCOMES

The following day about 4:00 PM I told my wife I wanted to have Proton Radiation Therapy at Loma Linda. The next morning I called the patient referral office to start the process of proton therapy. I canceled my appointment with the LRP doctor.

23

I mailed or faxed all medical history and other forms they sent to me. I received a letter about a week later informing me of my consultation schedule of February 22, 2007 with a doctor.

I feel extremely blessed to have been treated at Loma Linda Medical Center. What a wonderful group of people who are committed to serving God and people in their medical ministry in that place. I can't say enough about them and they have a real heart for what they do. God has been so good to me in providing me with what I believe is the finest treatment available for prostate cancer.

FAMILY, FRIENDS AND SUPPORT GROUPS

Family and friends played a big role by supporting me on my decision and during the treatments. Two of my daughter came and visited me in Loma Linda while on business trips to Southern California. The friends I made in Loma Linda were a big part of the treatment. I never will forget Mark from California, Doug from Virginia, Brian from Australia, Scott, Dave, and Bob from Washington, along with Hank from Arizona, and many more.

LIFE GOES ON

Three months later, we are on our last day of a visit to Maui. Thirteen of my family are here at Napili Village, including my sister and brother. We went snorkeling every day except Sunday when we went to Hana. The road has 600 curves and 54 bridges, and most are one-way. It was a 10-hour trip.

Life is pretty good!

Jim from Emmett, Idaho –
Proton Beam

HOW THE JOURNEY BEGAN

The first time I became aware that prostate cancer was a serious disease, was in 1997, when I retired to my farm in Emmett, Idaho. My next-door neighbor had just undergone prostate cancer surgery and a heart bypass, all within a two-month period. He had major doubts about surviving his ordeal. In subsequent months he kept me informed about his PSA tests.

This was the first time I became aware of what PSA was and its importance in monitoring prostate health. I continued to enjoy the retirement years, and each year I would receive an annual physical through Medicare. My major health concerns back then were high cholesterol and newly diagnosed Type II diabetes. I relied on my general practitioner to prescribe the tests and to interpret the results.

Life was good.

In October 2006 I went in to have blood drawn for my annual physical. The next day I received an urgent call from my doctor's office, asking for me to come in ASAP because my PSA was high. The lab test showed a PSA of 23. It is noteworthy that a digital rectal exam had showed nothing. Additionally, there had been no urinary tract problems, no frequent midnight trips to the john, and there were no erectile dysfunction problems that a little blue pill couldn't fix. An appointment was arranged with a urologist from Caldwell, Idaho who visited Emmett to see patients each Friday.

The urologist's digital rectal exam revealed nothing. I told him the lab must have made a mistake and requested another PSA test. When I asked what the implications of a 23 PSA reading were, he said that urologists use a velocity measurement to gauge how aggressive a cancer is. He said in my case he couldn't make an accurate determination because my general practitioner hadn't run a PSA for the past four years. As a precaution we set an appointment in his Caldwell office for an ultrasound and biopsy the following Monday.

When my urologist's nurse called me into ultrasound room on Monday morning, I couldn't wait to ask her what the new PSA results were. She didn't have them yet, and called the lab at the Emmett hospital to fax the results. The new PSA score was a 26. When she told me the results, the nurse said, "It's a good thing you're here."

NEXT STEPS

The biopsy I received that day was a never-to-be-forgotten experience. Seconds seemed like minutes, and minutes seemed like hours, and the spring-loaded needle cracked again and again -- twelve times in all. My urologist had explained that the ultrasound showed "something" in the seminal vesicles, so he took samples there as well.

My son Jim, who lives in Caldwell, joined my wife and me when it came time for yet another appointment with the urologist, to discuss the results of the biopsy. That discussion took place the following Wednesday. The pathologist's report showed cancer and a Gleason score of 7, we were advised.

The urologist set up a next-day appointment for a bone scan at the West Valley Hospital in Caldwell. So we made another trip back to the urologist in Caldwell to review the bone scan results on another date. My urologist had the radiologist's bone scan report in hand and read through it: No obvious sign of bone cancer! It was the first good news in weeks. However, there was one cloudy area in the pelvic area.

The radiologist went on to note that the patient (me) appeared to have a severe arthritic condition in his left wrist. I rolled-up my left sleeve and called my urologists attention to my Swiss army watch which I explained I had neglected to remove during the bone scan. The watch was the severe arthritic condition. We all had a tension-breaking laugh. A CAT scan was scheduled for the next day for a more in-depth exploration of the cloudy pelvic area.

The day after the CAT scan, we again convened in the urologist's office to review the results. The radiologist determined that the cloudy area was not cancer, but was the result of an old injury. I couldn't recall any specific injury to that area, but I had been knocked around a few times during my career as an underground miner, which may have been the cause.

Finally, some good news. I was just beat up, and didn't have cancer anywhere else.

Now we knew the scope of the problem; the cancer was in the prostate. The cancer was outside the prostate and had spread into the seminal vesicles, but the cancer had not spread to the bones.

What next?

Treatment Choices and Personal Outcomes

My urologist explained that he wouldn't recommend surgery since the cancer had spread outside the prostate and there was no assurance of total removal. Other alternatives, he explained, were radiation treatment and hormone treatment.

He explained that radiation would cause side effects and hormone treatment would not be a permanent fix but would buy some time and not cause any permanent side effects. We decided that hormone treatment with Lupron should begin immediately. I dropped my drawers and my prostate cancer treatment was underway.

The doctor also prescribed Casodex, which is a chemotherapy drug designed to kill cancer cells. Another PSA test and Lupron (hormone) injection was scheduled in four-months.

My wife and family were kept fully informed of the unfolding developments of my prostate cancer diagnosis. At this point in time, we were advised that the hormone treatment would probably buy us two years. I was extremely skeptical of radiation treatment, since my first wife had died of breast cancer after undergoing extensive treatment that only made her last days unbearable.

Also, my prostate cancer neighbor had suffered side effects from his radiation treatments that included a rigid, shrunken bladder that reduced his bladder capacity to about 8-ounces, and ended his sex life.

My next stop was the Internet of course, where the answers to any question you could ever imagine resides.

Entering "prostate cancer" in Google yielded a plethora of information. I spent days searching the various sites: John Hopkins, Sloan Kettering, Mayo Clinic, NCI, etc., etc. All of these sites provided good information, but nothing new unless you didn't mind having a few radioactive seeds wandering around in your body. Admittedly, I was becoming depressed and ready to accept my fate.

Then Divine Intervention took a hand!

My wife and I have been horse people for many years, but, as our bodies have become less resilient with age, we've gotten away from saddle riding and into harness driving, which is generally safer. One Sunday in early February 2007 my wife had gone to an arena in Nampa, Idaho where her (horse cart) driving club was holding an event. The arena was located fairly close to a lady who does quilting for my wife, so she brought some quilts along to drop off.

As my wife was leaving the quilter's home after a brief visit, she said, "I don't think I've seen you since my husband was diagnosed with prostate cancer."

The quilter immediately hugged my wife and said, "I'm going to give you a phone number. My neighbor just came back from prostate cancer treatment at Loma Linda and is now cancer-free."

Needless to say my wife could hardly wait to get home and call the phone number. We met with the man she called, a recently graduated Brother of Balloon, and his wife the next day and for the first time we learned that there was an alternative prostate cancer treatment that didn't cause all of the debilitating side effects that I'd heard about from cancer patients and read about on the Internet.

Once I knew to type the words "Loma Linda" into my Google Internet search engine, a whole new world of information on prostate cancer treatment became available. I quickly located the Brother of Balloon website, and ordered Bob Marckini's book about surviving prostate cancer, which had just been published.

I then emailed Loma Linda University Medical Center and requested information on their proton therapy program. From there, the decision was easy, and I arrived for my consult-pod-CAT scan session on April 23, went back to Idaho to pick up my wife, and returned to Loma Linda to begin treatment on May 7.

In early March 2007, before returning to Loma Linda for treatment, I went to the Emmett hospital to have blood drawn for a PSA test. This was just prior to my scheduled visit to the urologist for my second Lupron shot. The PSA reading was down to 0.14.

It is now amazing to think how I don't need to refer to the lab reports for these PSA numbers any longer. They are all permanently burned in my memory.

During the meeting with my Urologist, I explained to him how I had learned about Loma Linda and their proton therapy program, what their program consisted of, and the success stories of patients who had undergone treatment. My urologist sat silently as I told him that I was scheduled for a consultation and I planned to proceed with their treatment program. When I finished, he said, "I don't know much about their program, but I think you should go-for-it. I will provide copies of all your medical records or anything else they may need".

That pretty much brings my story to the present time, May 20, 2007, at the Creekside Court, 11067 San Juan St. Loma Linda, CA, which is an Oasis for Proton Therapy patients at LLUMC. I am telling my story at the request of a fellow patient who plans to publish a book relating the experiences of him and other patients.

Author's note: The answer to the questions of what role, if any, family, friends, support groups and/or humor played in this patient's treatment, and how things ultimately went, are still outstanding. Prostate cancer is a continuing journey. In future editions of this book, we will follow up on stories like this one, and provide the end for each story.

Elwood from College Place – Surgery, followed by Proton Beam

HOW THE JOURNEY BEGAN

My digital rectal exams started probably around the age of 45. In 1997, my PSA increased and my doctor decided to do a biopsy. This came back positive.

Being a Seventh-day Adventist, Proton Therapy at Loma Linda University Medical Center was known to me, but was not suggested by my doctor. I yielded to his suggestions and had a radical prostatectomy in October 1997.

Surgery went well and I was told that the cancer was encased within the prostate. Testing of lymph nodes did not show any spread. Several weeks following the surgery, on the morning after the requisite two-week catheter was removed, I found I was unable to urinate. I could not call the doctor until after 8 am. When I did get through, he said to come in and we drove to his office.

After waiting for around ten minutes of pure agony, the nurse took me in and said the doctor wanted a sonogram to see how full the bladder was, which I could have told them. After the sonogram, the nurse said, "Sir, I do believe that you are pregnant!"

After the nurse reported to the doctor, another catheter was inserted and immediate relief came. As for the other after-effects of the surgery, there was the normal loss of erections, but not of desire.

There were digital rectal exams and a PSA every six months for five years following surgery. The PSA went down to around 0.01. After five years the exam was changed to once a year. On about the eighth year, the doctor felt a small bump where the prostate had laid on the pelvis, prior to being surgically removed. Each succeeding check-up found the bump a little larger until September 1997, when I was told to come back in three months.

Three months later, the doctor said that we needed to do a biopsy of the nodule that had grown where the prostate had been. This was done in January, 2007 and it came back positive for cancer. In addition to that, my PSA score had climbed to 0.091. A test of the biopsy sample resulted in a Gleason Score of 8.

When the doctor received this report, he telephoned me, gave me the report, and explained my options:

1. Do nothing
2. Receive hormone treatment
3. Undergo radiation therapy

I told him I would talk it over with my wife and he gave me an appointment for the next Monday.

NEXT STEPS

It was somewhat somber around the house for a few days after we got the news. We told our son and daughter, but did not tell anyone else for several days. I made it a subject of prayer, as to which way to go. It was during one of these times, while resting, that the words Loma Linda flashed across my mind. I talked this over with my wife, and we decided going to Loma Linda was the way to go. I got on the computer, e-mailed Loma Linda and soon got a response back with information as to what they needed sent to them to determine if I qualified for the proton treatment that was offered there.

TREATMENT CHOICES AND PERSONAL OUTCOMES

When time came for the home town doctor's appointment and the subject of treatment came up, I informed him that my decision was to go to Loma Linda. He knew about Loma Linda through an acquaintance, who had also been his patient and had requested that his medical records be sent to Loma Linda.

The doctor was reluctantly cooperative, giving me the necessary bone scan and providing necessary records. The bone scan showed what they thought was bone cancer, so he ordered two MRI tests. After spending over two hours in the MRI machine, the verdict was that there was no bone cancer. Loma Linda wanted another test which was not available where we live, and that would mean going to Spokane or Seattle.

My doctor refused to send me for this test, so I had it done after arriving at Loma Linda for treatment. That test showed no spreading of the cancer to other parts around the tumor.

It was several days after we decided to travel to Loma Linda, California for treatment that we told the neighbors who would need to help watch over the house. Word got out soon to others, so I made it known also to my e-mail friends.

When my friends who were treated at Loma Linda got back from their ten weeks there, and told us of their experiences with the treatments and staff, we realized that we had made the right choice.

When I saw him for the last time before traveling to California, my doctor's final words to me were to make an appointment to see him in three months after I return.

FAMILY, FRIENDS AND SUPPORT GROUPS

Having gone through the experience of being told I had cancer once before, probably kept me from being distraught as before, but there was a little thought of why. But with the family promoting my decision on proton, and the assurance of prayers from family, pastors, church friends and others, I arrived at treatment knowing I would be in good hands and that what was supposed to happen, would happen.

After getting into the treatments and meeting others in the same condition, the friendship of the others in treatment promoted a very positive outlook while being treated.

Ron from Sacramento – Surgery

HOW THE JOURNEY BEGAN

At seven I was diagnosed with a heart murmur. It prevented me from participating in most sports until I was 13. At that point I had fallen in love….with basketball. I made a decision to take the problem head-on and play. Death was a risk I'd gladly take to play the sport I loved.

At 24, I developed gangrene, when a tissue that covers my stomach wrapped around something and died. I didn't find out until after the surgery how close to death I came.

At 40, it was Meineres, a disease with debilitating vertigo that leaves me progressively going deafer in my left ear. At 50, it was Type II diabetes, which I have been able to control so far with diet. Along the way, there have been broken bones, including a foot, leg (3 times), wrist, hand, collarbone, thumbs, fingers, along with torn stomach muscles and cortisone shots to knees, feet and shoulders.

And through all that, I still play volleyball at 57.

The point is that my body and I have always done battle. I view it almost like a competition. Tell me what I need to do to win and I'll give it my best shot, no matter the affliction. When I found out I had cancer, I realized my body was making its next serious attempt at the knock-out blow.

My doctor, who it turns out had a father who died of prostate cancer, believes in preventative medicine. One of the things he did was send me for yearly PSA tests when I turned 50, even though there were no symptoms. For the first few years everything was fine, and then my score jumped to an 8.

I went to a medical specialist who had gotten his degree around the same time the Constitution was signed, and never advanced his studies after that, apparently. The biopsy was extremely painful and I bled for six weeks after the procedure. The results came back with a suspicious quadrant that might have indicated cancer, but the doctor decided to take a wait-and-see approach. I was scheduled for another PSA six months later, and that came back as a six. Six months later I had a 4-something PSA, which was later followed by another that showed a slight rise.

I requested a different doctor and got a great one. He did another biopsy, which was virtually painless. The bleeding stopped in two to three days. The results of that biopsy came back the same as the first: a suspicious quadrant, more wait and see. A subsequent PSA showed another slight rise, to 7. When the third biopsy was done, we finally had confirmation. I had cancer.

NEXT STEPS

The doctor explained what I had and, rather than recommending treatment, he gave me a book and other reading materials. He suggested that we have an appointment in six weeks to discuss the options. I was off to the Internet, where I studied every kind of treatment I could find, researching the Internet endlessly, and looking at pictures I had never before wanted to see.

TREATMENT CHOICES AND PERSONAL OUTCOMES

I talked to my wife and we both reached the same conclusion: a radical prostate surgery was the option that would give me the best chance. I had a PSA of eight by this time, a Gleason Score of 6, and was 57 years old.

I think I deal with things differently than most people. I don't need pep talks. I don't need camaraderie. I view treatment for a disease as a competition: me vs. my body. One on One. Okay, may be it was two on one in this case. I did have a great doctor on my side.

One of the hardest things to deal with prior to the surgery was people who knew I had cancer, asking me how I was doing. I had no symptoms, no pain and I refused to focus on the treatment until we were close to the surgery date. My idea has always been that you don't want to get "up for the game too soon. You just want to be ready at game time. I'm very good at compartmentalizing and for 23.9 hours a day, my cancer just wasn't a part of my world… except for the "How are you doing?" questions.

When I was admitted to the hospital, I was mentally ready. I would approach the battle in segments. My first task was to live through the surgery. Because of the heart murmur, I had pre-prepared by having a series of heart tests that all checked out great.

It was good that we went through this, because my "normal" EKG looks like one for someone who's just had a heart attack. One time, an anesthesiologist almost cancelled my surgery for a hernia because of my odd EKG results.

When I woke up in the recovery room following surgery, I knew that I had won the first battle with my cancer.

I have an odd way of calming myself down in situations like these. I realized during my gangrene operation that if I died during surgery I would never know what happened anyway. Why get excited about it? Oddly, that thought seems to have a very calming effect on me. I know it probably doesn't work that way for most people, but it works for me.

My biggest fear going into the surgery was not the potential bad news of the prognosis, but rather the catheter that I would rely on for two weeks following surgery.

I was about 8 when my family visited my grandfather in the hospital. I noticed a tube with yellow fluid coming out from under the sheets. I asked my mom what it was and used the rest of my childhood to develop a deep-seated fear of catheters. That fear, which I acquired that day, has now grown to phobic proportions.

When I awoke from surgery, that catheter was the first thing I checked. I found it right where I expected it to be and was immediately queasy. That catheter became my main adversary in my battle to recover from the surgery.

My second focus in my battle with my body and cancer was the prognosis I would receive following surgery. I was immediately relieved when I talked with the doctor and he said the surgery was a success, that all of the cancer had been contained in my prostate, and that he felt they got all of it. He indicated that he was able to preserve all the nerves and that meant that "Mr. Happy" had a chance of being happy again, some day in the future.

Phase 3 of my battle was now upon me: getting mobile enough to leave the hospital. I was lucky. My surgery and the after-effects were virtually painless. I only used my pain medicine drip twice while I was in the hospital, and one of those times was for my back, which hurt from lying in bed so much.

If it was not for my catheter fixation, I might have been jogging around the hospital. Instead, I kept walks to the bare minimum because I was just grossed out to have the urethral catheter following me around everywhere I went. Mr. Happy wanted to go left, the catheter wanted to go right, and I wanted to go lay down for two weeks until it was out.

I will say that it really didn't hurt. The problem was 99% in my brain. However, it was my brain and my body that were waging this battle, and it seemed that I was fully committed to being a wimp about the long tube that went everywhere with me for that two weeks.

My next battle, as odd as it may sound, involved my intent to walk only enough to keep my lungs clear during the first two weeks I was home. This was because of the catheter that is a part of the first two weeks of recovery, following surgery, and how uncomfortable that thing is when you are moving around.

My wife aided and abetted me in achieving my goal. It was her care that got me through those weeks with a minimum of discomfort. She catered to my needs; brought me drinks, prepared my food and made deals with the local market to keep me stocked with diet root beer, which became my recreation and my obsession during that time.

I don't know if, when she married me at the tender age of seventeen, she realized that "For Better or Worse" would include emptying catheter bags, or applying cream in very personal places where the catheter chafed. I owe her a great deal for all that. I counted the days, one by one, until the catheter from hell would be removed and I could begin my recovery in earnest.

Once the catheter was removed, I increased my exercise measurably and to my displeasure, quickly regained the ten pounds I had lost immediately after surgery. The biggest problem I had during that time was the waistband of my pants rubbing on my surgical scar, but that was little enough to worry about. After only ten weeks, I was back playing volleyball.

LIFE GOES ON

For a time, I had a problem with incontinence, but after three days of that, I felt okay as long as I wasn't sneezing or rising from my chair suddenly. I had one naptime "oops" moment, which kept me in the diapers for the first week when I was sleeping, but the diapers were out of the equation for daytime use after two more days, and after a week, I was able to forego them at night. It wasn't long before my control was good enough for me to be able to go to the movies, although I always sat at the end of the row, just in case.

Sex was a big question on my mind before and after surgery, and I have to say that afterwards, the sex was weird. If anyone is thinking about prostate surgery, I would encourage them to read all they can about retrograde ejaculation.

In my case, "Mr. Happy" seemed semi–interested quickly, but to put it in an appropriate frame of reference: if you consider the sport of basketball, think of Mr. Happy as moving from being a center to a point guard. He's tall enough to play, but not quite in shape for a real game under the hoop. Dunking is out of the question, but on some days he can touch the rim.

Obsessing over the issue of sex probably didn't help the situation. Techniques and approaches had to change to make intimacy meaningful, and the climaxes became bizarre. The first time, I had to ask myself if I was done, and my answer was that I didn't know.

And then it got even weirder...

A climax that felt like it was going to be the real thing wasn't, and urine spurted out where semen used to be. It made a mess, definitely ruined the moment, and came as quite a shock. The experience sent me running back to the Internet, where I found out this was fairly common.

Why don't the doctors tell you about this?

I found that the weirdness eventually stopped, but it did happen three or four times. I seem to have a bit more control lately.

Hopefully, all this will settle down over time. After three months, I can fairly say that the sex is good enough to keep me from being horny all the time, but I'm still hoping for improvement. The doctor put me on some medicine to help with the erections, but that hasn't seemed to do much but cause a burning sensation in my nose, and who knows what that's related to?

In summary, the surgery wasn't very painful and went extremely well. I do suggest that you pick your doctor carefully. Who the doctor is can mean the difference between success and failure, and comfort and pain.

I never really felt like a cancer patient through the whole experience, since I had no symptoms and surgery did seem to go so well. I do suspect that the impact of being a cancer patient will settle in every time I have my PSA checked, and have to wait for the results.

Good luck and I wish you all well as my journey continues...

Paul from Augusta – Proton Beam

HOW THE JOURNEY BEGAN

In August of 2006, I went in for a physical exam. I was fifty-two at the time. Sometime during the previous two years, I had called in to the MD's office and left a message about getting a PSA done, since I had turned 50. I never received a call back. Now I wish I had been a little more aggressive about getting that done.

In September 2006, my first PSA came back as 5.0, and a referral was immediately set up with a urologist. That same month, the urologist did a Digital Rectal Exam and found nothing. He said we could either do another PSA test to confirm the first one and then a biopsy if it was still high, or we could go straight to the biopsy. I almost suggested dispensing with the second PSA and going straight to the biopsy, but kept my mouth shut. Like so many people my age, as a result of my upbringing, I wanted to believe that physicians are near-omniscient and always know what's best.

The next PSA came back as 5.7. I panicked. I thought that if it went up 0.7 in one month that could mean it wouldn't be long before it doubled, and that would be bad news.

In November, a biopsy was taken. I thought I counted the urologist taking ten samples, but it could have been twelve. After the biopsy, I was advised to call back the following Monday to get the results.

The following Monday I called, but found that the results were not in yet. I called back again over the next few days, only to find the results were still not in. Finally, on November 30, 2006 I called and, just as I dreaded, was told that the doctor wanted to talk to me. I got the next available appointment and, sweating bullets, waited for the MD to give me the bad news. There was a "small amount of cancer," he said, but they found it at an early stage.

As a sidebar: I have discovered that manually manipulating the prostate, as in the case of a digital rectal exam, can artificially raise the PSA for the next 3 days. I had my first two PSAs done at a lab within three days of having a digital rectal exam.

When I heard that I had cancer, I felt totally defeated. I felt like I'd played the game of life and lost – and lost big. I liken it to the feeling I had when losing a Little League baseball game. At that age, it's difficult for a boy to see past the immediate importance of a temporal event like a baseball game. At that age, especially when you're competitive, you get angry and disappointed with yourself, and with the opponent who won.

It felt the same with finding out I had cancer. It made a big dent in my self-image.

Whenever someone expressed concern over my situation, I wanted to scream, "So why don't you do something about it?" It didn't help when someone would come up to me and say, "You look good." It felt like they were treating me like a terminally ill patient, whom they wanted to make feel good, to think everything will be alright, even though they know that's not so.

An appointment was made for the Tuesday following the diagnosis to discuss treatment options. The urologist went over "all" the options that prostate patients have available, as well as the options that he felt were appropriate for me and those that were not. Included in the list were watchful waiting, hormone treatment, cryoablation, surgery, brachytherapy, and external beam radiation. Proton beam therapy, such as that offered at Loma Linda University Medical Center and a few other locations, was not mentioned.

My urologist indicated that surgery, brachytherapy and external beam radiation were appropriate for me, reviewed the side effects and, when I asked what he felt was the best of the three options he recommended surgery.

I sat there for a moment, chewing through the options, and almost let my natural inclination take over and go for the brachytherapy. When I say I almost let my natural inclination take over, I mean that I normally get the facts before me and make an immediate decision. I don't like to waste time. However, in this instance, I told the doctor that I was going to mull it over for a few days before I decided.

My wife has always been my number one cheerleader. I dreaded telling her that I had cancer when she came home from work that day. I knew that she would take it as a major blow when I told her. The whole time we've been married, I've always grieved anytime she has grieved. I never had anything but a superficial relationship with her mother, father or brother, so when her father, brother and mother died, the grief I experienced was more over the fact that my wife grieved, and not as much over the loss of her family members. I anticipated a similar experience as I waited for her to come home from work.

When she finally got home, we sat as I listened about her day. Afterward, I worked up the nerve to tell her that a small amount of cancer had been found in the prostate, to which she responded, "That's not good." It was a matter-of-fact response, but I knew that she was already grieving inside. I felt it, even though she is a master at masking negative emotions.

Of the people I told about my cancer who were Christians, all told me they would pray for me. Each time someone told me that, my emotional knees buckled. I know my voice cracked on a few occasions, and I know I at least cried on the inside. As I told people who were not believers, I found that some of them responded a bit more negatively than the believers. I did not tell anyone from my church until I had decided to have proton therapy and was already on the road to Loma Linda. I am not the sort of person who is comfortable with the fuss they tend to make over people when they get word of things like this. I just wanted to be off and on my way to dealing with it.

The response of people from my church has been more substantial than that of my non-church friends. I've received a large number of cards and letters while at Loma Linda. All the phone calls I've received have been from believers, with the exception of one.

NEXT STEPS

Once I received my diagnosis, the real investigation began.

Of course, the Internet was the major tool. Having access to information retrieval systems at a regional university where I work was also a blessing. In addition to looking at websites related to prostate cancer, I searched for the most recent peer-reviewed articles using the MEDLINE database. After a couple of days of research, I tentatively decided on brachytherapy as my treatment, but still felt like I should sit on it for a while longer. For a few days, no one knew about it except my wife. I did not immediately blurt it out to the whole world, but selectively mentioned it to some folks not in my everyday walk of life, but who had an important position in my life.

I decided not to tell my parents, both of whom were eighty-one years of age. I suspect that most people would think this was horrible, but my reasoning was that they would see cancer as the end of the road. My mother would likely not react as negatively as my father, but I think she would still be somewhat fatalistic about it.

I've heard my father say many times, "You can't beat cancer." I figured that if I did nothing I might outlive my parents anyway, so why inject this bit of grief into their last few years? Besides, because I caught the cancer early, I figured the chances were that I could beat it and go on with my life.

I did tell my brother and he's been very supportive, although I think he's not too sure how to interact with me on the subject.

Within two to three days after the diagnosis, I e-mailed a long-time college buddy and told him I had been diagnosed with prostate cancer and would be making a decision on treatment in the next few days. Ten minutes after I sent that e-mail, he called the house and told me that his father had gone to Loma Linda, California, to be treated for prostate cancer, and had tremendous success.

I remembered when his dad went to Loma Linda to be treated for prostate cancer, but I figured it was a treatment he could have received at home, but for some reason wanted to do it in Loma Linda. I'm not sure what I thought about it back then, but I also may have thought that maybe he was going there to get some weirdo treatment. Be it traditional treatment or weirdo treatment, I didn't make an effort to find out about it back then.

My friend suggested that I call his dad the next day. After my friend hung up, I immediately went online and searched on the terms "Loma Linda prostate cancer." I found the website for the Proton Treatment Center at Loma Linda University

Medical Center and decided that my tentative decision to go with brachytherapy was even more tentative, at least for a while.

The next day I called my friend's father and talked for about forty-five minutes. Everything he told me, I had already read online the night before. My phone visit with my friend's father seemed to confirm the need for more investigation. The next few days included a return to MEDLINE, where I found that everything I had read on the Loma Linda University Medical Center website was confirmed by peer-reviewed research.

I also e-mailed Bob Marckini, the founder of the Brotherhood of the Balloon, a prostate cancer support group. Bob encouraged me to include proton beam therapy in my list of considerations. At no time did he tell me to forget all the other options. He simply suggested that I read the testimony of Terry Wepsic on the ProtonBob website. That testimony turned out to be the most influential of all the input I received.

Terry is an oncologist who selected the treatment method for himself. It's one thing when a physician tells someone else that a treatment method is the most appropriate one, but when he selects it for himself, that speaks volumes. I was particularly impressed with the degree of detail Terry included when investigating his options, including a visit to the Seattle Prostate Institute, which is considered by many as the number one place in the world for brachytherapy. I saw no need to repeat Terry's investigative trek; I figured I would only come to the same conclusion.

I did not ask my urologist's opinion of proton beam therapy. If he didn't tell me about it because he didn't know anything about it, then he would have been in no position to offer an opinion on proton beam therapy. If he knew about proton beam therapy but did not tell me about it, then I considered that a potential lack of professionalism – and why would I want to deal with someone like that?

I didn't ask either of my primary care providers for their opinions, as I had already made up my mind by that point. One of the primary care providers asked how many patients had been treated at Loma Linda. I figure he was either trying to get me to think how prevalent the procedure had become, or he was trying to get updated himself; he indicated he knew nothing about proton beam therapy.

TREATMENT CHOICES AND PERSONAL OUTCOMES

Based on my research and discussions with others, I selected proton beam therapy as the treatment mode for me.

I travelled to Loma Linda University Medical Center (LLUMC) in Loma Linda, CA. I think my wife pretty much accepted my decision. She seems to defer to me when it comes to scientifically-related decisions, although I'm not sure that trust has always been warranted. In this one case, she may have had reservations but, if so, she hid them well.

One week after I made my decision, Bob Marckini e-mailed me and suggested that I obtain a copy of his book You Can Beat Prostate Cancer. Since I had already made my decision, I thought it overkill to purchase the book. A few days later I ordered the book anyway, thinking that it would help Brenda understand the procedure a little more thoroughly.

What I found when I read the book was that it is written for the layman. Bob takes all the complicated terminology and makes it palatable to anyone. I noticed that it has helped Brenda, which showed in the way she asked questions and conversed on the topic of prostate cancer.

The main side effect that I have had as a result of proton beam treatment has been increased urination at night. I'm not sure how much of this is because of the protons and how much is because of the 16 oz. of water that you have to drink before each treatment. I may have had some fatigue but, because of my regular aerobic and strength training exercise, it didn't occur or it was masked by the fatigue from the training.

Everyone at Loma Linda University Medical Center treated me wonderfully. I found no one who was unkind or showed any impatience with me. My physician was always ready to give all the time I needed during each appointment. That same sort of report is routinely provided by other patients when they talk about their physicians at Loma Linda. All the radiation techs seemed to look after me very well during my treatment.

I need to reiterate that my wife has been my number one cheerleader throughout the entire prostate cancer experience. She endured a lot while I was gone the nine weeks required for treatment. Then again, my wife has always put other people ahead of herself. Since, at the time of this writing, I have yet to return home, I can't yet comment on readjusting to home life.

Dr. Lynn Martell, a key person in the Loma Linda experience, mentioned during a Wednesday night support group meeting that Loma Linda University Medical Center was looking into how they could support spouses who must remain at home while their mate is away for treatment. I suggested to him that Loma Linda contact Seventh Day Adventist churches near the patient's hometown and have them offer to shepherd the spouse at home during the treatment time. I hope they do that. It could be the next big step in treating the "whole" person, which includes that patient's family.

FAMILY, FRIENDS AND SUPPORT GROUPS

I have been very well supported by my home church, First Baptist Church of North Augusta. During my treatment, I received a number of cards and a few phone calls from members of the church.

Before going to Loma Linda, I did not attend any prostate cancer support groups. I think the reason I didn't attend support groups while I was at home was because of pride;

not wanting to admit that I needed it. I wasn't comfortable talking about it, except with a few people.

After I arrived at Loma Linda, I opened up a bit more, and attended the regular Wednesday night support group meeting put on by the Medical Center, along with weekly Tuesday and Thursday evening potluck dinners for prostate cancer patients at the hospital.

I kept my sense of humor throughout treatment and anticipate I will do so throughout the return to normal life. Having somewhat of a sideline as a stand-up comedian, I suppose I might get some mileage out of the experience. Sometimes when I need to excuse myself to go to the bathroom, I might say, "My prostate's singin' a tune!" I suppose when I get back home people may ask if I brought back any souvenirs. I might respond with, "Yeah, a fried walnut!" referring to my prostate which was now shriveled up by the proton treatment.

LIFE GOES ON

This cancer thing has reinforced the fact that, no matter what, I'm not getting out of this life alive. It also reminded me of how important it is to be a good steward of the life and body God gave me. Pay attention to what you eat and don't eat. Pay attention to preventive medicine and don't skimp on the cost. I'm also reminded that at no time am I served positively by playing the role of a victim. Once you step into that mentality, it's too easy to blame others for your condition.

Taking charge of your medical care is ever so important. I was raised by parents who looked at physicians as practically omniscient. Whatever they said was the gospel. Now I can see the basis of their statement, "He's a good doctor", when referring to any of the physicians they ever used. Anytime they said that, it was because of the way the physician interacted with them on a personal basis. I don't think the doctor's medical skill ever played a part in their evaluation of physicians. It was based solely on whether they liked him as a person. My parents assumed that just because a person was an MD, that person knew all there was to know about any medical condition, and if the doctor told them they should do a certain thing, they believed it.

That upbringing carried over with me well into my adult years. My own experience with cancer has demonstrated to me that I need to be more vigilant over my choices when it comes to treatment, and maybe even skeptical about what I'm told. If not skeptical, at least I need to be cautious when receiving information provided by a physician.

This cancer thing also drove home the fact that I believe that if a person has no personal relationship with Jesus Christ, he doesn't have much to lean on while he goes through all this stuff. I would encourage all those folks who have been skeptical of "all that Christian stuff" to re-evaluate their perceptions. Trying to measure-up, trying to do good deeds in order to win God's favor isn't what it's all about.

Joe from Westminster – Proton Beam

HOW THE JOURNEY BEGAN

My journey started in April, 2004, but I did not recognize it at that time. I was having a routine well-adult visit with my internist when out of the blue, he started talking to me about prostate cancer. Lots of men get it, and I was approaching the age when it becomes a concern. It is normally very slow-moving, and in my opinion, treatment options are not necessarily good. The cancer can be treated, but the quality of life can deteriorate substantially.

My physician indicated that in many cases the treatment is worse that the cure, and watchful waiting can be a prudent step. He indicated he had debated this approach on more than one occasion with the urologists at The University of Colorado Health Science Center and felt strongly. My PSA at the time was 3.3, and had risen from 1.9 three years earlier. The results of my digital rectal exam were normal.

Two years later, in May, 2006, my PSA had risen to 4.8, while my digital rectal exam remained normal. My internist recommended a visit to the urologist, which I did.

Based on test results and a normal digital rectal exam, the urologist indicated that my choices were to have a biopsy or wait six months and check the PSA again. I chose to wait. Both my doctor and the urologist indicated that the likelihood of cancer under these conditions was twenty to twenty-five percent. I chose to believe that with only a one out of four chance that I had cancer, that I was cancer free. On the other hand, my wife was convinced that I had cancer and being a librarian, she did extensive research on possible causes, treatments and outcomes.

As it turned out, she was right.

In January 2007, my PSA was 5.3, and the digital rectal exam was again normal. Given the rise in PSA, it was time for an ultrasound (normal) and a twelve core biopsy. After the biopsy, I was instructed to call the urologist, which I did on February 8, 2007. He advised me that five of the twelve biopsy samples were positive for cancer. I had scheduled an appointment with my doctor for five days later to review treatment options.

My reaction to the diagnosis was pretty stoic. "OK," I thought. "I have cancer. There are no symptoms and I feel fine, so now we have the time to start the process to determine how to move forward."

Next Steps

Research, that's what I did.

When I first saw the urologist in the summer of 2006, my wife did extensive Internet research. She found volumes on information on possible causes and a variety of treatments for prostate cancer. Much of it was conflicting, even between what appeared on what were considered to be knowledgeable, authoritative websites.

In October 2006, I found a piece of paper with the e-mail address of an old friend from Colorado, whom we had lost touch with. He responded immediately and noted that he had changed to a new e-mail address and the old one was going to expire within the week. Had that happened, we would not have renewed our connection and I would have missed some very important information.

In December, we received a Christmas e-mail from Joe. In it, he related his incredibly positive experience of being diagnosed with prostate cancer and being treated with proton beam therapy at Loma Linda University Medical Center. This was the first we had heard of proton therapy or Loma Linda.

When I received the confirmation that I had cancer, I contacted Joe, and he spent a significant amount of time explaining proton therapy, his experience at Loma Linda, and his research. He pointed me toward the Brotherhood of the Balloon website, and more information about the Loma Linda Proton Center.

From this point on, research became considerably easier. In all the prior research my wife had done, she had not discovered proton beam therapy. Yet once she had the terms down and the understood the Internet links, the research came together easily. The more research we did, the more we came away with the feeling that the outcome from proton beam therapy would be as good as the other treatment alternatives, but that the incidence and likelihood of short- and long-term side effects was significantly less than from the other treatment choices. And it was non-invasive.

Next was a visit to my urologist

By the time we met with the urologist, we were 95% certain that proton was the way to go. Our goals for our meeting with the urologist were to:

- Fully understand the findings

- Understand the treatment options from the urologist's perspective

- Understand the urologist's recommendations

- Determine if there was any evidence or findings presented by the urologist that would change the path we were following.

The urologist explained the PSA and biopsy test findings and then went into detail outlining all of the treatment options, as he understood them. Proton beam therapy was not on his list.

When I asked his recommendation, his response was that I would be fine with surgery, Brachytherapy, or external (conventional) beam radiation. I then asked him why he had not mentioned PBT and he responded that it:

- Was not available in Colorado

- Was more expensive

- Was just another form of radiation.

I thanked him for his information and indicated that we would review the options and three books he had given us to read.

The books were helpful in the sense that they clearly outlined the invasiveness of the recommended treatments and the associated side effects, to the point that they helped us continue to move in the direction of proton beam therapy.

The next step was to set up a meeting with my internist on February 22 and review my options one final time. When we met, I outlined the findings, recommendations from the urologist, and that I was leaning heavily toward Loma Linda and proton beam therapy. At that point he excused himself and then returned with a printout of the NCCN (National Comprehensive Cancer Network) Clinical Practice Guidelines in Oncology for Prostate Cancer. He reviewed these in detail and noted that:

1) the recommendations from the urologist were dead on with the guidelines

2) Proton beam therapy was not listed as a treatment.

I responded with study summaries and reports from the Loma Linda site that showed patient outcomes as well as side effect rates of proton therapy, compared with the other treatments.

In the end, while he did not recommend that I pursue proton therapy, he did say that he wanted to raise it as a topic within his local cancer consortium. He indicated that he would support my decision and asked me to keep him advised of my progress.

After we met with the urologist, I called the contact name that Joe had given me at Loma Linda. The person was friendly, open and knowledgeable. After a short conversation dealing with my status and numbers, I was requested to send my documents to the hospital for screening. These were faxed the next day, and within a week, I received word that my file had been reviewed, the insurance company had been contacted and that I was covered. The next step was the scheduling of my consultation. It was that easy!

When I initially received confirmation of my diagnosis, I advised my manager and local human resources representative at work. Both gave me their support. After the meeting with the urologist we told our kids, ages 25 and 22. I think it was a sobering time for both of them, but by this time we were in a position to speak positively of the treatment plan we were pursuing.

After the initial consultation at Loma Linda, when I was accepted into the program and the treatment schedule was established, we told other relatives, friends and co-workers. The hardest part was to convince them that I felt great, had no symptoms and have an excellent prognosis.

There have been interesting discussions with friends. Some are knowledgeable about things like PSA scores, and have annual check-ups. A few others do not. I have taken on a role to bring them up to speed and convince them that they need to monitor their PSA's and become more knowledgeable about prostate cancer.

TREATMENT CHOICES AND PERSONAL OUTCOMES

As of writing this, I am halfway through my treatment at Loma Linda; twenty-two treatments down and twenty-two to go. I have had no side effects. The people, both the staff and the other patients, are great. The atmosphere is incredibly supportive and in the words of Dr. Lynn Martell of Loma Linda, "None of us got here by accident". We all feel blessed.

FAMILY, FRIENDS AND SUPPORT GROUPS

Here at Loma Linda, I am participating in the activities offered for patients, such as potlucks, the Wednesday support meeting, dinners out with the group, the exercise at the Drayson Fitness Center. In every case, there is lots of discussion about how we all got here.

I have been sending bi-weekly e-mails to family, friends and co-workers, keeping them updated on my progress. I am also sending these to both my internist and to the urologist.

LIFE GOES ON

I think this has brought my wife and me closer together. I also feel compelled to spread the word to others on the benefits of proton beam therapy and Loma Linda.

Dr. Robert from Pittsburgh – External Beam Radiation

How the Journey Began

I was diagnosed 9-1/2 years ago at age 70. An increase in my PSA (5.9) led to a biopsy by a urologist. The diagnosis was delivered to me via a dinner-hour telephone call; a miserable, inconsiderate way to communicate with a patient.

The physician asked me to call his office the next day to schedule a visit and discuss surgery. I was obviously distraught, and extremely upset and nervous. Within a day I started calling some friends to seek advice on which treatment process they selected. I started to share the situation with family and close friends. Then, as I calmed down, I laid out a strategy to seek information on treatment options, side effects of treatment, time involved in recovery, etc.

NEXT STEPS

Visits were scheduled with seven physicians over the next couple of months (3 more urologists, 2 radiation oncologists, and a medical oncologist, family physician) to seek alternative opinions. I also called all of the relevant health organizations (American Cancer Society, National Cancer Institute, etc.) for materials and publications to obtain a background. UsTOO, the prostate cancer support group, was brought to my attention by a former work colleague who was treated, and I started to attend chapter meetings to share the views of other patients.

One radiation oncologist took me aside at a group meeting and indicated that it really did not matter which treatment I elected. All appeared to have the same outcome. I also called a former neighbor who is a prominent medical oncologist with a substantial research background and asked his opinion. He referred me to a radiation oncologist with whom he worked and indicated that this was the person he would personally use if he had to deal with his own prostate cancer. I carried my biopsy slides with me as I visited the various physicians.

We then went off for a year end vacation in London and Paris. What better place to make a decision? I essentially made up my mind on the treatment in Paris.

TREATMENT CHOICES AND PERSONAL OUTCOMES

I elected 3-dimensional conformal radiation at the University of Pittsburgh Medical Center (UPMC) with the prominent radiation oncologist recommended by my former neighbor. This was preceded by a couple of weeks of Lupron shots and Casodex. The shots were administered through a prominent UPMC medical oncologist. I had to stop the Casodex due to a very unfavorable reaction.

The radiation was set up on a 7-week schedule, 5 days per week at 8:00 am so that I had the day free to go about my professional life. The staff at the radiation facility at UPMC was particularly considerate and helpful. Side effects were minimal and did not alter my life; they mainly included fatigue and some bowel irritation and urinary urgency. The side effects faded quickly when treatments were completed.

FAMILY, FRIENDS AND SUPPORT GROUPS

I continued to attend UsTOO support group chapter meetings at two local hospitals (UPMC and Allegheny General), and read a great deal of material on prostate cancer treatments, side effects, long term prognosis, etc. Candidly, I was somewhat psychologically depressed by the strain, uncertainty of the future, the impotence brought on by the treatment (which faded in time). I spoke with several friends who were diagnosed shortly after my situation unfolded, providing them with the information I had gathered. One selected the same treatment, two selected alternate treatments (surgery, and brachytherapy/seeding).

LIFE GOES ON

The impact of the cancer has affected me psychologically, and I have become a little overly sensitive to every ache and pain (I call them the ache and pain of the week). I do follow-up with the radiation oncologist twice a year, and a medical oncologist 3 or 4 times a year.

My professional life was really not impacted (I am a Professor of Communications) and I continued to meet my students and work obligations; a year later I took my class to Germany for a special Spring Break program.

Richard from Ft. Lauderdale – Proton Beam

How the Journey Began

A high PSA (5.5) was detected during an annual physical in September 2006. It took a while to get a urologist to see me, but I had a second blood test measuring free PSA to confirm the first test. I then had a 10 point biopsy and was diagnosed in February 2007. My Gleason was 6, and my Clinical Stage was diagnosed as T1c.

Next Steps, Treatment Choices and Personal Outcomes

My first call was to a friend and mentor from my active duty days (Coast Guard - 34 years). The first words out of his mouth were Bob Marckini. As a result, my first treatment decision was proton beam therapy. This occurred after I read Bob's Marckini's book.

After sitting down with my urologist, my second treatment decision was traditional surgery. After doing some more research, my third treatment decision was robotic surgery. I reviewed dozens of individual treatment descriptions and found lots of good information at UsTOO and other online sources.

I did some traditional research in the medical library at the university where I teach, and read several books. I finally ended back up where I started: proton beam therapy.

FAMILY, FRIENDS AND SUPPORT GROUPS

I had a lot of support through this process, and got a lot of information from people who were kind enough to tell me when they were diagnosed with cancer, and what they did. Doctors (I met with an oncology radiologist in addition to my urologist) tended to see the world through the porthole of their specialty. I talked to several on the phone, including a radiologist from San Diego, who did the proton thing.

Family friends provide a lot of support and information. The information ranged from traditional to far out in left field.

I was not shy about telling others about my situation. I felt a need to return the candor of others who helped me so much on my journey.

LIFE GOES ON

The following are some philosophies and quotes that that inspired me:

1. All cancers are different; all patients are different
2. The best treatment for you is the one you believe in after doing due diligence in research.

I am a survivor in the making

Unity is strength.

Knowledge is power.

Attitude is everything.

"I adopted the notion of **carpe vitam**. That means 'seize life.' That's my motto: seizing life. Life and all of its meaning and its richness came to be for me what I'm all about and how I want to live." Mortimer Brown, 79 years old, 4 year survivor of colorectal cancer.

"When thinking won't cure fear, action will." William Clement Stone

"You have to be the CEO of your own care." Greg Ferris, Navy Seal, 31 years old, battling leukemia

Come to the edge, He said.
They said: We are afraid.
Come to the edge, He said.
They came. He pushed them,
And they flew . . .
                              --Guillaume Apollinaire

"Have every teenage girl lose her hair for six months, and she'll be a much better person." Amy Dilbeck, a 23 year-old bone cancer survivor for 7 years.

"A positive attitude towards treatment was a better predictor of response to treatment than was the severity of the disease." (From Getting Well Again, by Simonton and Creighton)

John from Minnesota –
Undecided Treatment

How the Journey Began

When I retired five years ago this past May, I had visions of writing about tall tales of adventures like sailing around the world, or walking the Appalachian Trail, or just pedaling my bike across the country. Instead, I find myself on a different kind of journey, with PC, and by that I don't mean political correctness. I write because if a little medical hangar flying can help someone avoid some of my mistakes it will be worth it.

My journey starts in December, 2003.

Knowing and doing are not the same. I know I need to see a dentist periodically, and eventually I do. I know I need to monitor my cholesterol, and after having a heart attack, I really pay attention to what my numbers are. I know that one of the things you should do is have the old colon looked at and so I scheduled myself for a sygmoidoscopy that December.

After the flex sig procedure, everything was fine except that my proctologist said he could feel something on my prostate. I didn't know he would be checking that part of my anatomy, but since he wasn't charging extra, I figured it was a "pilot good deal". He said I needed to see a urologist ASAP and that there was a good one in the same building. He gave me a name.

What a coincidence! I had an appointment with that very same doctor later in the month. Also, this particular urologist had been recommended to me several years earlier by an internist I was seeing at the time. He was also listed perennially as a "Top-Doc" in the Minneapolis/St. Paul magazine and turned out to be very friendly and personable. I figured I would be in excellent hands to evaluate what was going on with my nodule.

NEXT STEPS

I started preparing myself for the likelihood that I would need a biopsy, something I felt was akin to getting shot with a gun, only the bullets were smaller. Let's see: You are going to place a large object where the sun doesn't shine, to shoot a hollow needle through the wall of my rectum and into my prostate, tearing flesh and capillaries and maybe even veins and who knows what else along the way, to extract a few cells. I started to imagine what a biopsy needle must look like on the scale of my poor little prostate.

I put away my irrational fears and kept my appointment. But before that, I had my PSA checked; another thing you should do, like getting your cholesterol checked, and about as much fun. With both tests, you feel so much better after it is over if the numbers are in the green range.

I have been told that starting at about age 50, (earlier if you are at increased risk), all good little boys should have their PSA checked. My previous PSA for a flight physical had come back at 0.77, with anything zero to four considered normal. I took great pleasure in my number, as I figured I had the PSA of a teenager, even if other things didn't quite work like a teenager's does. In fact, that is why I had scheduled myself with the urologist. Things were no longer working like a young race horse and I found it more and more necessary to assume the old-man position on trips to the little boy's room.

Blood was drawn two days before my visit for the PSA test. The appointed hour came. I was ready for anything, even a biopsy. After the usual small talk, I was told my PSA came back as 0.44, I knew it, still just like a teenager. Any lower and I would be pre-puberty.

Finally, the moment came for the finger-wave, the digital rectal exam, and boy did it hurt when he felt the nodule that my proctologist had first noticed. The next thing I heard was: "Well, your PSA is so low, I think I'll put you on a course of antibiotics, and we will check everything in six months."

"Thanks doc," I said. "I'm out of here. No biopsy is fine with me."

Six months later, we went through the same drill again, except my PSA was now 0.62. Hey, that's still below my previous high of 0.77. I opted to wait another six months, which turned into a year and a half after visits from Hurricane Ivan the Terrible, and Katrina. For those who don't live in Sunny Florida, those were a string of hurricanes that did a lot of damage, including to my place. I got wrapped up in repairing my leaking roof and missed my next appointment in Minnesota and didn't schedule another until January, 2006. After all, at that point the appointments were still routine. There was no need to hit the panic button.

I knew that it is not how large the PSA number is that counts, but how your PSA numbers change over time. If you see a doubling, or even just a 0.75 rise in a short period of time, it is worth getting checked out. My PSA came back that January at 0.32 -- a 50% reduction. With numbers like that, I now felt I was bullet-proof and had avoided the dreaded biopsy. My urologist did not expect to see a PSA that low either. I didn't know what was going on, but felt that certainly it couldn't be cancer. I went back to Florida to continue working on the hurricane damage.

In August, we returned to Minnesota to await the arrival of grandchild number five. In September, it was back to the proctologist for the full treatment this time. Coming out of sedation after the colonoscopy, he told me that he had felt a very large nodule on my prostate and that I really needed to see someone.

Not long after that, while visiting my daughter in the hospital and my new grandson, I had an event that totally got my attention big time. During a trip to the hospital men's room, I saw blood where a man doesn't ever expect to see blood. My urologist was in the office complex next to the hospital and I beat a path to his office.

I'll never forget trying to explain to the young female receptionist why I wanted to see my urologist without an appointment, or at least be able to speak with him. No matter how I pleaded with her, she was not going to call him or help me. I finally got to him by calling his home and asking his wife to have him call, which he eventually did. He explained that the bleeding was possible for a number of reasons and not to worry unless it didn't stop, and for me to see him in a few days. By this point, I wanted a biopsy regardless of what my PSA numbers were, which for that visit turned out to be 0.54, or eight points below my June, 2004 number.

The biopsy finally took place January 15, 2007 and on the 19th, after playing phone tag with my urologist for several days, I learned that I had prostate cancer throughout the right side of my prostate gland. Further, the biopsy came back as a Gleason of seven.

A Gleason Grade is derived by looking at the morphology (shape, structure, color, and pattern) of the cancer cells compared to normal cells. There are two patterns, with possible values between 1 and 5, which comprise a Gleason Grade. The first number is the primary pattern and the other number is the secondary pattern. There are other subtleties to a Gleason Grade, but mine was calculated as 4 + 3, or seven. That meant the primary pattern in my case was not good and can only be one number higher, hence a fairly serious case of PC.

Nothing quite focuses one's mind like being told you have prostate cancer. I have learned a lot since that January date. Most importantly, I learned that you want to catch this stuff early, while it is still confined to the prostate to have the best chance of survival.

While I am not on the backside of the power curve yet, I'm close.

To go over some of what I think were my mistakes along the way:

1. In spite of my urologist being recommended by two doctors and being very friendly, he turned out not to be a good choice for me. During my office visits over the last several years, I began to feel that we were not connecting as we should. For one, I would ask him what the aging male can expect when it comes to ejaculate volume. I could definitely tell something was changing in that department. He never answered that or other questions that would have told me what is normal and what isn't.

   The cancer was profuse in half my prostate, so what I was noticing makes perfect sense in hindsight as half the gland was no longer functioning. My big mistake here was that I didn't listen to my inner voice and instead stuck with this doc because I liked him.

   There were also other problems, as well. In the beginning, I was never apprised of the need not to stimulate the prostate with an ejaculation for 3 days before drawing blood for a PSA test, because it skews the numbers. That also goes for mechanical stimulation like a Digital Rectal Exam (DRE) or riding a bike or anything else that could stimulate the prostate. In my case, this did not explain my very low PSA numbers. Still, it is part of the protocol when drawing blood for a PSA test.

2. The biopsy is not quite the dreaded procedure that I envisioned. It is uncomfortable, to say the least. However, it is bearable, and at this time it is the best way to really tell if you have prostate cancer for sure. You shouldn't let yourself be put off like I was.

3. I feel I should have had a biopsy after that first visit, even when my PSA was 0.44. I have since learned that an abnormally rising PSA trend, or a high PSA number, or an abnormal DRE are sufficient reasons to have a biopsy. I also learned later that my urologist was an optimist (his words), which explains why he didn't order a biopsy on my first visit as he felt it surely had to be something else.

4. My health was more important than fixing hurricane damage. It is all too easy to get swept up in what seem like important things at the moment and let routine medical tests languish.

5. Here is what I consider to be the most important thing I should pass on: Low PSA numbers like mine don't give you a free pass. Though rare, there are a number of reasons that your PSA doesn't go up when you have prostate cancer. All along I felt something was not right with the "experience" or the plumbing, but got hung up on my low PSA numbers. This was a very big mistake, especially when I had an abnormal DRE. I guess that makes me an optimist also.

6. After seeing blood, what I went through in order to talk to my urologist was further confirmation that I was with the wrong doctor in the wrong group. I have a theory that attitudes and sensitivity like I encountered that day start at the top and flow down hill.

So, an adventure begins for me that I didn't want. However, I am not alone.

It is estimated 218,000 men will be diagnosed with prostate cancer this year, rising to over 300,000 per year in the coming decade. Roughly, 30% of men will end up with prostate cancer by some estimates. That's over 1 in 5. Prostate cancer will probably become the number one cause of death for men due to cancer. Lung cancer is number one now, but that should change as more men stop smoking.

Here are two other startling facts I didn't know: More men get prostate cancer than women get breast cancer, and if that is not bad enough, more men will die from prostate cancer than women will die from breast cancer. Yet, breast cancer receives the lion's share of attention and research funding. That needs to change, not by taking money away from breast cancer research, but by providing more money for prostate cancer research. Hopefully, it will.

There is another thing about prostate cancer that makes it unique. You can end up having to pick your own treatment. I have learned that there are several ways to treat PC, all of which work fairly well if the cancer is still confined to the prostate and none of which work very well if the cancer has escaped. Hence the very important need to catch it early. My next step is deciding which treatment is right for me.

Please note that nothing I have said should be construed as giving medical advice. My comments should not be interpreted as specific medical advice and should only serve as nonspecific background information. Consulting a qualified (not me) medical professional is always best.

This journey continues…

Russell from Vermont – Proton Beam

How the Journey Began

I was diagnosed the end of October 2006, after a visit to my primary care physician. He found that my PSA had risen from 2 to 4.2 in just 6 months, so he thought I should have a biopsy.

The biopsy showed that I had prostate cancer with a Gleason score of 7. The doctor called my wife and said he wanted to see us in his office by 11 am that morning. He gave us the news, and it was a shock.

You are never ready for someone to tell you have cancer.

The doctor said he was concerned that it was outside the prostate because of the back pain I was experiencing. He ordered a bone scan and a cat scan. They showed I had arthritis of the spine and that the cancer looked to be contained within the prostate.

He then proceeded to make me an appointment with a radiologist, but I would have to wait almost 4 weeks to see him. When we arrived for that appointment at Dartmouth Hitchcock Medical Center in Hanover, NH, we were directed to the doctor's office. When he arrived, he said he would have to review my file because he had not looked at it before then. He took a few minutes, and then said he didn't know why we were sent to him, and that we needed to see the surgeon first. He then proceeded to tell us our options for radiation or seeds, and made an appointment for us with a surgeon and for an MRI.

The appointment was made for December 22 for the MRI, and January for the surgeon. I had my MRI and the doctor said he would call Friday before Christmas with results to let us know whether it was outside the prostate or not. They never called until after Christmas. Needless to say, our Christmas was a very emotional one for me and my family. We were sure it was bad news and that the doctor didn't want to tell us till after Christmas. We all prayed and left it in God's hands.

My wife and I have been married for 47 years, have three wonderful children along with their mates, and ten grandchildren that are even more wonderful. We both have much to live for.

That Monday after Christmas, I got a hold of the doctor and he said the MRI looked good and the cancer was contained, but felt we should do something right away. On January 2, 2007, we met with the surgeon. When he came into the office with us, he told us he had not had a chance to look at my file yet. We waited while he looked at the file, and then he informed us that he couldn't really talk with us today about it because the pathology slides were not in the file and he had to find out where they were. He said he would review my file the next Thursday with a group of other doctors. In the meantime he set up a surgery date for me for Feb 5, 2007. He said they would call on Friday to set up an appointment to see him again. We never did get that call.

After the appointment with the surgeon, we left for Florida to deliver a trailer, and on our way there we received a call from a friend in Alabama. He told us of a fellow who had gone to someplace in California and said he would have him call us. His name was Bill and the next day we received a call from him.

Bill told us all about Loma Linda proton beam therapy treatments he had received. Awhile back, the receptionist in our doctor's office overheard us talking about Loma Linda, and she told us she knew of a patient that had gone to Loma Linda. She could not give his name to us because of patient confidentiality, but would call him that evening and have him call us. That night he called us.

His name was Albert, from Norwich, who was an engineering professor at the college in our town. Both he and his wife talked to us at great length. By the time we got off phone we knew for sure what we were going to do, and learned that they had stayed at Loma Linda Springs Apartments, where we ultimately stayed for my treatment.

NEXT STEPS

My wife proceeded to do research on her handheld computer all the way to Florida, during our trip with the trailer. We then called Massachusetts General first, because it was closest to us and we were told that they had a proton treatment center there. When we called, we couldn't find anyone there that could help us and they didn't even try to find anyone who could help us. We then called Strands Hospital in Jacksonville, FL, where we received the same response.

Next, we put a call through to Loma Linda Hospital in Loma Linda, Calf. We reached the receptionist first and asked to talk to someone about proton beam therapy, and were put through to a girl named Brooke immediately. Before my wife got off the phone with Brooke, we knew all about the treatment and what we needed to send her to get the ball rolling.

My wife immediately called our doctor's office and had them fax records to Loma Linda. We were on our way.

The next few days, we were back and forth on the phone with Brooke at Loma Linda. My wife called our family doctor and told him what we were thinking of. He said he didn't know much about it, but would do some research over the weekend and wanted to see us on Monday when we returned from our trip.

That Monday we met with him and he said it was our decision and that he didn't know if it was good or bad. We told him we had already made up our minds to go and he gave us his blessing.

Our consultation was set up for February 27, 2007 at Loma Linda. We were in Florida when we left for there.

We drove out on Route 10 all the way, and it was a very good trip. We had our first appointment on the 27th and my treatment pod made on the 28th. They gave me a two week start date, which was better than they had said it would be. When we were traveling across the country, our doctor's assistant called and said it would be a wait of at least a month to six weeks. We told her that would be a real hardship, as we were already driving there. We both had left full-time jobs for the treatment.

She said for us to pray about it and she would too and see what could be done. That blew our minds because we never would have been told to pray about anything back home in our hospital.

Treatment Choices and Personal Outcomes

We chose the proton beam therapy and they said it would take 44 treatments to complete my care. It was the best choice we ever made.

Our family was very supportive of our decision and they were all praying for us. We never realized how many people cared until "we" got cancer. I say we because it does affect both husband and wife.

In talking with so many of our friends, we were surprised to learn how many have had prostate cancer and the many different ways to treat it. In talking to so many there were so many bad side effects that we felt the proton beam was our best choice.

LIFE GOES ON

Our lives have dramatically changed since we first learned of the cancer. We have taken a close look at what's really important in our lives, and realized how much God has blessed us, and how important our family is to us.

We have exercised six days a week since we came to Loma Linda for treatment and have never felt better. We have grown in our spiritual lives. Realizing that this life is only temporary and that there is eternal life through Jesus Christ our Lord was something we knew before, but which came home with more reality than ever before.

Dr. Lynn Martel of Loma Linda was right when he once said during a support group meeting that we do praise God for our getting cancer. It truly is the best thing that ever happened to us, for the way it changed our lives for the better.

Our stay in Loma Linda was been unbelievable. We were anxious to return home, but will take our experience here with us.

Loma Linda seems like it is surrounded by God's angels. The whole town has a certain quality about it that one cannot find elsewhere. What more can I say? I am returning home a whole man in every way.

As we get back home, we know that we will do what we can to spread the word to others so that they may have the same experience we have had.

William of Coal Valley – Brachytherapy

How the Journey Began

I was born to a family of twelve children: 6 males and 6 females. As our father got into his 70s back in the early 1970s, he found he was experiencing some back pains. A check with the doctor suggested surgery to find the problem. Once the surgery started, they found he was in late-stage cancer, and were not able to identify what kind of cancer it was.

Several years later, in the mid 1980s, my oldest brother was experiencing blood in his urine. After the doctor checked him out, he was put on antibiotics, which cleared up the problem. The doctor indicated that he thought there might be another problem as well, but didn't elaborate on his thoughts. Six months later, my brother was diagnosed with advanced prostate cancer. He survived several more years, dying before his 65th birthday.

As a result of my brother's cancer, my two other older brothers went to Mayo Clinic to get checked and found they both had prostate cancer. They each had surgery in 1990. Their physician recommended that I get my PSA checked annually due to the family history. One of the brothers that had a radical prostectomy had a recurrence and died before he was 69.

I had three years of PSA readings and my PSA values stayed constant, around 1.7. In 1994 my PSA values jumped to 2.4. I went to a urologist and requested a biopsy. He wasn't sure why I wanted a biopsy since my PSA readings were below the guidelines that he used, which indicate that a PSA of 4.0 was acceptable. I informed him that I had monitored my PSA readings for the last three years, and since I was a product assurance specialist by trade and thought in terms of trends and anomalies, I just naturally watched for a change in the PSA that would indicate that something might be happening. I considered my prostate to be like a machined part, like those I routinely inspect, and while being processed any variability in the testing and tolerance readings would indicate something was happening.

The result was that I was diagnosed with early stage prostate cancer. My Gleason score was 2-3, or 5. My PSA was 2.4.

NEXT STEPS

The only information or literature I could get was from the American Cancer Society, which was very limited. I also got some help from my brothers, which was also limited, being based on their personal experience with surgery. I was not happy with some of the side effects they were having and wanted to get more information on what procedures were available other than surgery.

Prior to going to the urologist to hear what my results were, I had talked to a brother-in-law who lived in Florida and talked about my interest in a relatively new procedure called brachytherapy. He knew of a lawyer who had brachytherapy several years prior and was more than willing to discuss the procedure with me. I received a call from the lawyer and our discussion lasted for an hour. He made sure

I knew that I needed to know what my Gleason Score was. I obtained all this information prior to a visit with the doctor regarding my biopsy analysis.

TREATMENT CHOICES AND PERSONAL OUTCOMES

I elected to have brachytherapy since I was told that there would be minimal side effects after treatment. Initially, my brothers felt I should have the same thing they had. After I had the treatment, which was on a Thursday, I was back playing golf on Monday. I received excellent treatment from the doctors and staff of the radiation department where I was treated. The nurse who worked with brachytherapy patients was excellent and responded to any request for information regarding possible complications. My wife Sandra was very supportive and concerned with all aspects of my treatment recovery.

FAMILY, FRIENDS AND SUPPORT GROUPS

There were no support groups available in my region to talk with regarding choices of treatment and/or side effects that may occur. I was always willing to share with family, friends, or individuals that wanted to know what option I had selected and why I selected it. Because of my family history, I was not dumbfounded by having prostate cancer. Knowing how it affected my family, I considered myself very fortunate to have had a father and brothers that I learned from.

I was fortunate to be able to talk to another patient who'd had brachytherapy six months prior to me, and was having great results and minimal side effects. He was also a golfer and had a hole-in-one shortly after his treatment. So when I went to get my procedure done, before they put me out, I asked the doctor when I was going to get my hole-in-one. They were laughing while I was going to sleep.

LIFE GOES ON

I had been retired for two years when I found I had prostate cancer. Because of my inability to find information or someone to talk to about their treatment options and/or side effects, good and bad, I contacted the American Cancer Society to get a prostate cancer support group started in my area. We have a total population of over 350,000 people in the Quad Cities area, which is located next to the Mississippi River between Iowa and Illinois.

We started out with five men and their wives in our group, and have grown to over seven hundred members. We have an excellent rapport with all the urologists in the area and attend numerous health fairs, handing out literature on the need for men to get an annual PSA test, and digital rectal exam. We also conduct seminars on prostate cancer.

Our support group affiliated with UsTOO International, Inc. in 1997 as an UsTOO Chapter, and I am the Senior Regional Director for seven states. I am now on the Board of Directors for UsTOO International, Inc.

I have spent the last 13 years working with prostate cancer patients and their families, assisting them in getting whatever information they feel they need to make a sound decision on treatment choice. I feel it is better for prostate cancer patients to research all the options that are available and talk with other survivors about the outcome of their treatment choice, so they can make a decision on a treatment choice based on knowledge and not fear.

Walter from the Villages – External Beam Radiation

HOW THE JOURNEY BEGAN

When I was turning 50 years old (I am now 65), my wife insisted I attend a prostate cancer screening session at Roper Hospital in Charleston, SC. There were several hundred men in the audience in an evening session that started at about 6 pm. The program consisted of doctors in urology, radiation, surgery, and pharmacology explaining everything you always wanted to know about prostate cancer. They also outlined every possible treatment then known (in 1991). At about 8 pm we all got a free rectal exam (DRE) from one of the 8 to 10 urologists in attendance. The doctor I had for the examination had been one of the leaders of the presentation and I liked his candor and easy manner.

Over the years, I was examined by him yearly with both a DRE and PSA tests. I had a PSA level that would go up and down but always stayed in the 2.0 to 2.8 range. When I turned 60, we both decided that twice a year exams would be wise, since I was gradually creeping up on the PSA level. When it would drop, it would go down to a higher level than where it started.

When we moved to Florida in 2005, my doctor told me to find a doctor here and transferred my records. At that point, my PSA was inching up over 3.0 and my new urologist started 3-month tests. Last October I hit a 4.8 (a jump from 3.8), so we did a biopsy. My staging was a T1c, with a Gleason of 3+3, or 6.

I had an appointment with the doctor with my wife, Barbara, in attendance. He told me, very matter-of-factly that I had prostate cancer. I was not surprised at all nor was I shocked or frightened. My previous doctor had told me years ago that this would probably happen because of the roller coaster PSA values. He had also told me for years that surgery should be the last option I should consider, depending on the severity of the biopsy results.

My new doctor went on to explain about the options that he felt I had. He suggested surgery using the Da Vinci robot, which he had done for some time. He also said that I could do seed implant with him doing the surgery and a radiologist doing the actual implantation. In addition, he outlined radiation and explained that I was almost a perfect candidate and he gave me a referral to a radiation oncologist who also does seed implant. He said to think, take my time, see about radiation, and generally figure out what I wanted to do. It was now mid-December 2006 and I decided I would see the oncologist immediately and decide after the first of the year.

We live in a retirement community of 65,000 plus people who are extremely active. Our neighborhood is very close and friendly. I told friends when I went for the biopsy and told them of the results. I have never felt any kind of shyness or shame about having prostate cancer, or that I wouldn't be able to handle it when it came. It seemed to me to be just something I had.

Four guys on my street had had prostate cancer – all but one had it surgically removed, the other had seeds 10 years ago – and all had had problems with severe side effects.

NEXT STEPS

After talking with the oncologist, I was tending toward seed implantation. He explained that he places his seeds on the outside of the prostate rather than the inside, because he feels he can direct their concentration much better and there is less risk of losing one or two into the urethra, etc. He also said that I also had the option of just doing 41 sessions of IMRT and that I was a perfect candidate for this treatment with my stage, my Gleason, and the percentage of involvement of my prostate.

At this point, Barbara and I started doing web searches and investigation. We also called Barb's cousin, who put us on to UsTOO, the prostate cancer support group, and all that its web site had to offer.

We read books, we talked to guys who had been treated, and we looked at the chat rooms on the UsTOO sites for surgery and seeds. I learned about the side effects that I was told were temporary that became all too permanent. Barb and I decided the quality of life after prostate cancer was important and we decided on full IMRT for 41 sessions.

TREATMENT CHOICES AND PERSONAL OUTCOMES

IMRT started in mid-January after CT scans and fitting of the leg frame, etc. The radiation center in The Villages is one of five locations of the Robert Boissoneault Oncology Institute. Their main office is in Ocala, FL and my doctor comes to The Villages every Wednesday. I met with him, or the residents, weekly for discussions on whatever was on my mind.

I had five sessions a week at 9:30 am, which lasted about 25 minutes. The actual sessions were run by a rotating team of five techs that really took care of me, were considerate, and just a joy to be with. All were in their 30's and 40's, had a good sense of humor and perspective, and never made me feel anything other than very positive.

After a few weeks of radiation, I developed a large boil on my butt just above the rectum. It was on the inside of the crack of the right cheek but soon grew outward so that it was uncomfortable to sit and walk for long periods. The head was about the size of a quarter but the whole thing was really big. The oncologist suspended the treatment for a week, put me on heavy antibiotics, and a super powerful ointment that worked well. I started treatments again as the boil got smaller and it was soon gone.

The biggest test seemed to come from the water I had to drink every morning. It involved about 20 to 25 ounces of water that I would start drinking at about 8:50 am, when we drove to the center for treatment. I had already had a cup of coffee and a bowl of cereal and it was hard to fit it in. In the beginning, I could hold this well through the treatment. As the sessions progressed, however, I found I could not hold the water as long and that I was always feeling that I might let go any minute. Flomax helped but it never handled the heavy pressure during the sessions. Twice I had to call for help and one of the techs held a bottle for me to relieve the pressure. I was embarrassed that they had to do that but they quickly helped me to get over that and we'd joke about it later.

The people I dealt with directly were wonderful – the rest of the staff was distant, almost to the point of ignoring Barbara and me. I think they didn't want to put a personal face on people or get involved with their lives and cancers – there were people there that were just barely hanging on with brain tumors, etc. I think this was their way of staying out of the tragedy before them. The techs used humor and an upbeat attitude to help me along. If they had problems coping, I wasn't aware of it.

Barb was with me every day at the center. She swabbed ointment on my butt, and generally followed my lead on moods, etc. We tried sex a few times and it wasn't as good as usual, and about halfway through treatment I began to feel fatigue in the afternoons or early evening that precluded anything but sleep. I was taking piano lessons weekly and stopped those because I just couldn't get up for practice.

FAMILY, FRIENDS AND SUPPORT GROUPS

I am a very positive person. At no time did I consider prostate cancer to be life-threatening or incurable. At the very least, I would die of something else before it got me. Humor is the very heart of my day-to-day existence. Barb and I see the humor in everything we do, we say, we see, we feel. We are incredibly in tune with each other so there isn't much we don't discuss with each other.

For that matter, I am not inhibited about talking about the treatment and its various effects to friends, family, neighbors, etc. I feel that what I go through is part of the human condition and I don't find that very embarrassing. Having UsTOO on my e-mail daily was wonderful. Their humorous e-mails were so silly and fun that I wound up forwarding the jokes to relatives, friends, and neighbors. I also had all sorts of offers of aid in transportation, prescription filling, etc. from neighbors on my street. That was very positive and I guess my keeping them informed on a regular basis helped us all feel we were a part of the treatment.

UsTOO provided answers for Barb that came up in the chat rooms. She would read questions and answers from people that would give her insights that I missed sometimes. The radiation center did not provide a real level of support for spouses, etc., that I think should have been there. Fortunately, Barb and I have such a close relationship that the lack of support on one end we provided for each other when needed.

LIFE GOES ON

Not much changed in my life. I am not at all religious and although friends said they were praying for me, I thought it made them feel better than it did me. If anything, I guess I've slowed down. I was a person that always had to be doing something. I no longer feel that need to be out and about. I never had much patience for fools and now I have no patience for people who seem to take things too seriously, who find crisis is everything. I seem to be questioning rules I used to take for granted of late, also.

All in all, the whole experience has not been terrible or life-altering to any great degree. I knew I would be okay after everything was finished. I also know that most men do not have an experience even remotely similar to mine and that I have been very fortunate. I now know that the very best thing happened 15 years ago when my wife nagged me to go to the prostate cancer screening and started me on the journey. Early detection and having a track record on PSA was the key.

A side note. In 1996, I got a cancer insurance policy that cost me approximately $400 a year. In the past 5 months, the insurance company has paid me nearly $20,000.00 in supplemental payments to handle out-of-pocket expenses. I tell every person I meet that is of an age who would find benefit in this unbelievable protection to investigate cancer insurance.

Jim from Olympia – Surgery, External Beam Radiation, Androgen Deprivation

HOW THE JOURNEY BEGAN

In 1989, I decided to help out the school district and get a bus driver license so I could back the school buses onto the ferry to get them serviced on the mainland. I was the district superintendent of schools on an island in the Pacific Northwest. We all pitch in to help when you live in a small school district. Besides, I had driven truck for many years and felt very comfortable driving a school bus.

As part of the licensing requirements I was required to take a physical. I had not had a physical since college and was a very healthy 50 years-old. At the doctor's office my wife asked that they perform all tests appropriate for a 50 year-old. It included blood draws for a number of tests. He stated that there was a new blood test for prostate cancer and would do that test as well.

Well, he called to ask us to come to his office to see the results of the tests. Everything was great, just like I expected. But he said the PSA was 39 and he would have to check to see what that means. The next day he said I should make an appointment with a urologist on the mainland to have a digital rectal examination. He suggested an experienced urologist who he knew personally.

The urologist found a firm spot on the prostate and said I needed a biopsy to see if I had prostate cancer. The notification that I had prostate cancer came over the phone.

NEXT STEPS

In 1989, there was no easy access to current information about prostate cancer. Visits to the library uncovered a few older books, so we started our journey to find out what options were available to me. My wife and I talked to our urologist who said, "Surgery is the gold standard" and he was ready and willing to perform the surgery. He was aware of the nerve-sparing techniques developed by Dr. Walsh. He said I was young, strong, and healthy so I should come through the surgery in fine shape.

Back in 1989, the only other option available to me was external beam radiation. My wife and I met with a radiation oncologist who explained the process and was willing to give us the names of men who had radiation. We heard of damaged bowels, incontinence, erectile dysfunction, and burned skin. We were not able to find reliable data about survival benefits.

Watchful waiting was not mentioned. The message from the medical professionals was to get the cancer out of you or destroy it where it lies.

TREATMENT CHOICES AND PERSONAL OUTCOMES

During our reading we connected with books written by Bernie Siegel, <u>Love, Medicine, and Miracles</u> and <u>Peace, Love, and Healing.</u> We agreed that we are Mind, Body, and Spirit, and that we wanted a doctor who would treat the whole person, not just the body part. I asked every doctor that treated me if they had read Bernie's books and if they believe in treating the whole person. I did not want a "body part" specialist working on me. All parts of my body are connected and my mind and spirit are a huge influence on my total life and healing.

The words "Gold Standard" rang loud and clear in our minds. The urologist had performed hundreds of radical prostatectomies and had successfully spared the nerves on his patients. He explained that if the cancer had spread to the nerve bundles he would remove the cancer and thus destroy the nerves controlling an erection. He mentioned that dead men don't have erections, so getting the cancer out was the top priority.

I was informed of the importance of Kegel exercises to strengthen my sphincter muscles so I would remain continent. I faithfully performed the exercises, even stopping urination mid-stream to make sure I had the muscle tone necessary. It was a good message as it worked for me.

I was also given the choice of storing my blood for the surgery as it was described as a very bloody surgery. If I did not, I would expect to get blood from a donor. It was an easy task to go to the hospital and donate a pint of blood to myself. The three pints of blood would be stored and made available for the surgery. I was very glad that I did, as the surgeon used all of the stored blood.

Recovery was quite easy. I expected to be worse off than I was. I left the hospital in three days and was walking around with the catheter dangling the next day. I knew getting up and walking around was important to getting my body to heal. It did. I was continent five days after the catheter was removed. That was very empowering.

After a few months of watching my PSA my urologist called to let me know my PSA did not drop as low as it should.

There must have been some cancer that escaped the gland. The lymph node biopsy from the surgery was negative.

The urologist then suggested that I see a radiation oncologist and go through 35 sessions of external beam radiation to destroy any prostate cancer cells left behind from the surgery. I made arrangements to catch a ferry to drive to the radiation clinic on the mainland for five days a week for seven weeks. The radiation was a piece of cake. The major stress was catching a ferry, driving to the clinic, driving back to the ferry, waiting in line, and finally getting home. It took a lot of the romance out of island living. I had no negative side effects of radiation. I got tired of getting undressed and dressed so I always wore comfortable clothes and joked a lot with the staff. It has always been important for me to keep a sense of humor through difficult times.

But, six months later my PSA only went down to 0.2 and started to increase. I was told that my two major treatments had failed to get rid of the cancer. According to the statistics available I would have from 1 to 3 years to live, so I better get my life in order. I guess I still don't have my life in order, as it's been 18 years since my surgery.

As my PSA continued to rise, I began charting them. I kept asking when to start androgen deprivation therapy (ADT). No one came up with a definitive answer. When I read that once prostate cancer no longer responds to androgen deprivation there was no other option but chemotherapy and chemotherapy may have a survival benefit of less than three months.

I began ADT when my PSA got to my "panic point". I asked everyone I knew when to start ADT and the answer came from Dr. Susan Slovan when she said there is no approved protocol for when to begin ADT and if you decide to do intermittent ADT you need to again define your "panic point". Therefore I began ADT when my PSA was 49 and watched it go down every month. It went down rapidly. I stayed on ADT for over a year and my PSA went to the lowest point it had been after surgery and radiation; 0.2. I stayed on ADT for almost another year and then decided to go off treatment.

I have been doing intermittent ADT for over seven years but now I chart my testosterone level as well. If ADT is supposed to lower testosterone, we should have a measure of it every month to see if it works. I had to convince my doctor to get the testosterone test along with my PSA.

When I go on ADT my PSA goes down and my testosterone went from 350 to 17. It was working. I have raised my "panic point" to a PSA of 20 before I go back onto treatment.

My goal is to keep my prostate cancer dependent on testosterone as long as I can.

When I meet with prostate cancer researchers I challenge them to find out why prostate cancer becomes androgen independent and find a way to stop it from doing so. If we could keep prostate cancer dependent on testosterone, prostate cancer could become a chronic disease because ADT works.

At an FDA hearing for a drug to treat advanced prostate cancer, Dr. Mark Moyad said, "There has only been one drug approved for advanced prostate cancer in the past 40 years, and that's taxotere, a chemotherapy drug."

FAMILY, FRIENDS AND SUPPORT GROUPS

My wife was at my side through the whole process. We discovered that prostate cancer is a family disease. She attended every medical appointment with me, which was a true blessing. Because of our selective hearing, we found that she heard things that I didn't and I heard things she didn't. We also learned to take a tape recorder along because our memories are never as good as the actual recording. If a doctor refused to have the session taped, we would find another doctor. I respect her knowledge and ability to see through the medical language to see the impact on my total being and on us.

I learned about some prostate cancer support groups eighty miles from my home. I attended a number of them and found that I was not alone and that many men have found ways to improve the quality of their lives, despite prostate cancer. I heard men say, "I may have cancer, but cancer does not have me!" Others said "prostate cancer does not define who I am" and "I can live WITH prostate cancer". It was so encouraging to meet men who had been dealing with prostate cancer for a number of years and were leading productive, happy lives. Their lives changed, but they learned to adjust and appreciate living.

LIFE GOES ON

Unfortunately I also found out the subtle ways a person with cancer can be discriminated against. I took it upon myself to spread the word about prostate cancer, back in 1989, when there was very little awareness of the disease that was killing 40,000 men each year. I spoke at state conferences and told everyone I knew that they should get screened. I really feel the screening and early treatment saved my life. I was almost evangelistic about spreading the word.

At the same time I was leaving my position and was applying for another school superintendent position. To make a long story short, I got very few responses from my applications and when I did talk to someone they always said, "Well hi Jim, how are you feeling?" I had a few interviews and they all ended with that question. It was obvious that my evangelism carried far and wide and everyone knew I had cancer.

I eventually applied out of state, where no one knew me. The first application resulted in an interview and contract. I did not offer the information about my cancer. There was a remarkable difference in how I was treated.

I went through the ethical dilemma of whether or not I should tell my school board. I was feeling great and the cancer did not hinder my ability to do my job. I talked with my wife and we decided to not say anything.

This went on for years. I never talked about it and my wife and I kept our "little secret". Remember, this was eighteen years ago. The public was not well informed about prostate cancer and the word "cancer" was equated with death. I know it was very hard on my wife as she had no one to talk to about her concerns. I was getting quarterly PSA's and watched the numbers increase slightly every time.

By this time there was information on the Internet and more public awareness because of organizations like UsTOO, International, and the American Cancer Society. Prostate cancer was being talked about, though not openly. This began the next stage in my treatment.

My wife and I read a lot about the power of the mind and a positive attitude. We read books and even took some courses on guided imagery, the power of the mind to image health and healing. We also read a great deal about diet and exercise as it relates to cancer. I began an exercise program that involved calisthenics, weights, and cardio exercise. I faithfully exercise for an hour every other day.

We also changed our diet to a primarily vegetarian diet and followed the recommendations of Drs. Snuffy Myers and Andrew Weill. It is important to follow a heart healthy diet and to exercise to keep the whole body healthy.

Then came the day my secretary come to me very upset. Her husband had been diagnosed with prostate cancer and she was sure he was going to die. I could not keep my secret any longer. I asked if I could meet with the two of them. It was quite a relief to finally "come out of the closet" and talk about my experience with prostate cancer. I felt I could be an inspiration to him, as his PSA was just above average. When I told them my PSA had been 39 they both gulped. I also told them that I had been treated with surgery and radiation and I was living a very normal life as far as anyone could see.

When I saw what this knowledge did for them I realized that many men and their families could benefit from my experiences. I decided it was time to tell my school board first. Then I could go public about my cancer.

I was so inspired that I started a support group for men and their wives to discuss surviving prostate cancer. I took training from ACS and my wife and I got trained to train other support group leaders. It was a great feeling. People were coming out of the woodwork to tell me their experiences and to share with others. Men were no longer alone and their partners also had someone to talk with.

A large part of my healing is the benefit I derive from helping others deal with their disease. I attend UsTOO chapter meeting across the country and facilitate a group in Olympia. I have become an officer in UsTOO, International and spend a great deal of time helping develop new chapters and responding to calls about prostate cancer. The "thank you" messages I receive give me energy and encouragement to continue dedicating my time and energy to helping my brothers.

I now see every day as a GIFT, to be opened like a present and thankful for the opportunity to live another day. You see the world differently when you realize that you have a limited number of days on earth. Love is the greatest gift to give and to receive. My greatest joy is being able to help others.

Dealing with Your Prostate Cancer

If you have read or purchased this book, there is a good chance that you or someone close to you has been diagnosed with prostate cancer. If that is the case, know that there are literally millions of others out there who have wrestled with the disease and come out on top. In each of those cases, the messages have been clear:

1. The person who has the cancer is in charge of their treatment. No one should make any decisions for them about the nature and form that their treatment.

2. The physician is the patient's best friend as he fights for his life against prostate cancer. That being said, physicians are generally aware of those treatment options that they have been exposed to. A urologist is a surgeon and can generally be relied up to recommend surgery, because they know and trust surgery. A radiation oncologist will likely have a lot of faith and confidence in radiation therapy. General practitioners will generally be aware of the sorts of treatment that their network of peers espouses. There are

several additional handfuls of treatment options beyond those options that the average health care professional will not be aware of, each of which promises a successful outcome and varying degrees of impact on the patient's quality of life. From that, it follows that...

3. It is the patient's job to locate the available treatment opportunities and sort out his options.

4. The patient must be a warrior in the battle against prostate cancer. As in the case of Jim from Olympia, a terminal diagnosis is only one physician's opinion. Eighteen years later, Jim can attest to the fact that there are options that can save a man's life, and all should be considered and potentially used. It is up to the patient to carry that battle forward.

Good luck with your battle against prostate cancer, whether it is you who leads that very personal battle or if you are rooting from the sidelines. Remember that, in spite of our gender's apparent unwillingness to talk about prostate cancer, there are many voices in the Prostate Underground who are waiting to be heard, if only you ask the question.